Published by:
Association of Reflexologists Ltd
Victoria House
Victoria Street
Taunton
Somerset
TA1 3FA

+44 (0)1823 351010
www.aor.org.uk

Printed in the United Kingdom.

ISBN: 978-0-9933909-1-3

Print run:
2 3 4 5 6 7 8 9 10   22 21 20 19 18

Contents

About the Authors

Tracey Smith FMAR BSc (Hons)

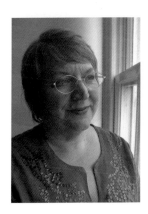

Tracey Smith is the Reflexology and Research Manager at the Association of Reflexologists (AoR). Tracey holds a BSc (Hons) in Immunology; she is a Fellow of the Association of Reflexologists has been a practising reflexologist for nearly 20 years, prior to which she was a scientist. Tracey originally joined the AoR to increase understanding and acceptance of reflexology through research. Moving reflexology forwards through the understanding and dissemination of evidence is very important to her.

Tracey is a regular speaker at conferences, has written reflexology articles and published scientific papers. She has also co-authored a number of AoR books and guides, including A Guide for Reflexologists: Healthy Ageing and Stress: A Reflexologist's Guide.

Sally Earlam FMAR BSc PGCE

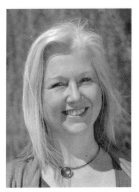

Sally qualified as a reflexologist in 1999 and is a Fellow member of the Association of Reflexologists. Sally has worked for the AoR since 2012. She was Head of Training and Education for 10 years and now works on a consultancy basis as their Senior Programme Manager. She has had a huge amount of experience including being a Board member for the Reflexology in Europe Network and was on the Profession Specific Board of the CNHC. Sally has been involved in teaching Anatomy and Physiology for many years, both as a qualified nurse and also as a reflexology tutor. Sally has co-authored a number of AoR guides and books including Supporting Conception and Maternity, Hand Reflexology , Reflexology for Menopause and supporting stress, anxiety and depression.

Laura Franzen MAR BA (Hons)

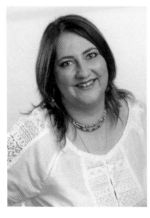

Laura is a Fellow member of the Association of Reflexologists and has been practising reflexology since 2012. She is fully trained in a number of renowned reflexology techniques, as well as in several other complementary therapies. In 2022, she gained a Diploma in Adapting Complementary Therapies for Cancer and Supportive Care from the world-famous Christie NHS Trust Integrative Therapies Training Unit.

She currently works as the Complementary Therapy Coordinator for St Margaret's Hospice Care covering the West of Somerset. Laura coordinates and provides complementary therapy treatments as part of the clinical team for patients and carers. When not working at the Hospice, she runs her own private practice in central Taunton, called Victoria House Therapies.

Sue Ricks HMAR

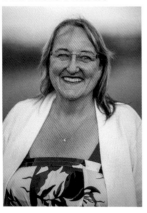

Sue Ricks is the founder of Gentle Touch Reflexology and has been working passionately in support of reflexology both in the UK where she lives and also internationally. She has dedicated herself to helping people of all ages to have access to reflexology through teaching, clinic practice and creating products and courses that aim to transform, help and educate. Sue has developed a speciality program of using reflexology for assisting babies, children and parents and has taught in schools, organisations and hospitals.

Throughout her career Sue has developed and refined her understanding and instinctual knowledge of the relationship between emotions and the human body.

Sue assisted the setting up of the Holistic and complementary therapies course at the university where she lectured in reflexology at the University of Derby. She is also the author of 4 books including *The Gentle Touch of Reflexology for Babies and Children*, a number of DVD's and teaching aids including charts. Sue is passionate about reflexology and the loving therapy that this is. She has interviewed a number of reflexologists from around the world that can be found at www.suericks.com/interviews

Sue continues with her Gentle Touch Reflexology, life coaching, mentoring and teaching and passing on the metaphysical meanings behind illness and disease.

Sue's website is www.suericks.com

Jane Sheehan HMAR

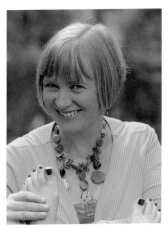

Jane Sheehan is the UK's leading foot reader - she reads personality traits in the shape and form of feet and toes. Jane qualified as a reflexologist in 1999 and after four years of practising reflexology and foot reading in her spare time, Jane left her nine-to-five office job and embarked on a career centred on her foot reading skills around the world.

Jane makes regular TV appearances (ITV's This Morning and "It Takes Two" the BBC's Strictly Come Dancing chat show in the UK, The Afternoon Show on RTE in Ireland, Sama TV in Dubai, Inside San Diego and Fox in the Morning in California and Channel 9 in Australia). She is also the author of several books: *'Let's Read Our Feet!'* is now on its second edition and is also available as an e-book and as a portable guide; *'The Foot Reading Coach'* explains how foot reading can be used as a tool for self improvement for everyone and her most recent book, *'Sole Trader – The Holistic Therapy Business Handbook'*, is based on her own experiences in setting up her successful international business.

Her website is www.footreading.com.

Introduction

As reflexology practitioners, we are mostly taught the intricacies of hard skin or palpable imbalances of a reflex in terms of a physical problem that is likely to be manifesting. Too often we forget that an individual is not simply a collection of past and present physical problems, but a swirling mixture of past and present emotional issues as well. Generally, we are usually good at considering all the physical aspects, but often neglect the emotional ones. By not taking the emotions into account and by not fully embracing their whole being, we are doing our clients a disservice which could cause needless anxiety.

We do also need to remember that reflexology is very subtle and any imbalances found need to be handled carefully and with great sensitivity. How often have you heard of clients having attended a 'reflexologist' and being told that there was something wrong with their heart or kidneys? This sort of statement causes unnecessary concern and worry - we need to be extremely careful how we approach such issues and how we support our clients.

On finding a reflex that is imbalanced, it's important to always consider the physical condition first since this will take us to the next step in understanding what is really going on emotionally and spiritually.

- Do they have a related illness now?

- Have they had a related illness in the past? No matter how long past, reflexology theory suggests that energy imbalances can be held in the tissues.

- Is there an issue with another reflex in the same zone that might be blocking energy in that reflex? E.g. if there is tension in the shoulder you may find tension all along zone 5, often in the knee and hip.

If none of these fit the situation, which is possible, then the emotion behind the reflex can provide invaluable insight into a potential reason behind that imbalance. By taking a look at the emotions and gently questioning your client along these lines, even though they may not immediately identify a link, after a period of reflection they are likely to 'get it'! Once acknowledged, detrimental emotions can be released over a timeframe that suits the client and dramatic changes in their health and wellbeing are more than likely to be the result.

It is of course believed that reflexology has been around for thousands of years in the Far East, yet in the West it is still relatively young at less than one hundred years old. The investigation of the emotions behind a reflex is even more in its infancy. You may read differing views in different books and just as there are different foot maps and different reflexology sequences, there is no right and wrong. For the emotional aspects, this book contains ideas from two well-known foot readers. They read from two separate modalities so whilst they don't always agree with each other's interpretation, we feel offering a choice of how to read will give you the opportunity to explore, experiment and benchmark for yourself. We hope that what they have found and shared helps to add a further dimension of knowledge to your practice.

We also wish to recognise that the physical pathologies come largely from the Complete Pathologies for Complementary Therapies book by Essential Training Solutions. We offer them our sincere thanks for allowing us to use their compiled information.

We hope you enjoy this book.

Tracey Smith, Sally Earlam, Laura Franzen, Sue Ricks and Jane Sheehan

The role of the reflexologist

This book is intended to guide you through the potential physiology behind an out of balance reflex point but also it indicates potentially tied up emotions too. Your training as a reflexologist is sufficient to allow you to understand the emotions that might be involved with a reflex, but you need to recognise that in working with these blockages an emotional release of some sort may result. Initially this may not sit comfortably with the way you work, but the emotional interpretation does not necessarily have to be shared with your client – it could simply be helpful for you to understand. As you become more comfortable with the concept you might want to start to explain to your clients that there is a school of 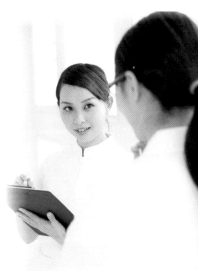 thought that links blocked reflexes to the emotions, and see where that goes with each particular client. The next step would be to explore gently to see if your client believes that they might have a block in that particular area. Of course this has to be handled very carefully and with great sensitivity, because as a reflexologist you are not a counsellor. Eventually you might feel that actually you want learn further about how to help your clients work through their emotionally complex issues, in which case there are many excellent courses in counselling available.

Often we choose to become reflexologists because we have a strong desire to 'help', and in helping others something within us is nurtured too. This strong desire to help can sometimes mean that, in our enthusiasm and without any intention of doing so, we almost cross the boundaries of other areas beyond reflexology. The obvious boundary we can cross in reflexology is that of the diagnostic role – referring what we find in the feet to physical problems. This suggestion is acceptable if we are referring to past problems, a reflex can be out of balance because of a past accident/ or illness. But if we start to pronounce that an out of balance reflex point means there is a problem or there WILL be an issue in the future, this is diagnosis and we all know that we cannot diagnose and should not be overstepping that mark.

When it comes to the emotions we have to be doubly careful for all sorts of reasons. Therapeutic touch and empathic listening can produce different reactions in different people and as reflexologists we have to be able to cope with those responses if we are going to help our clients release them. Support and empathic listening used to be the role of close family and friends, but as the world has become less orientated around the family nucleus and more fractured across the globe, this type of support has become less available. Also many people are very time short so multi-tasking with both fantastic reflexology and some supportive listening (even if only for part of the appointment) is becoming very popular. This means our role can, at times, come dangerously close to overlapping that of a counsellor. We have to recognise that this can happen and therefore we need to take baby steps when entering our client's emotional zone.

Reflexology is an intuitive therapy which the client's body reacts to, and will on the whole, tend to release a package of emotions just big enough for that person to cope with on that day. The release usually happens when the client is feeling safe – which could be in their own bedroom with the door shut tight or conversely with a group of supportive friends in the middle of a busy restaurant. It's where the individual feels protected and this may also be when they are with you in your treatment room, which is why it can be a good idea to have a box of tissues handy for those occasions. Tears are also something that if you are going to be aware of the emotions, you will need to prepared for. They're not predictable so you can't necessarily be primed for when they come, but when they do you need to have an idea of what to say. My favourite comment when this happens is simply - 'It's OK, let it go, you are in a safe place so just release' and to pass the tissues. It's has happened many times in the past and I expect it to do so in the future. Release of tears is a good step to letting that particular emotion go. However, we must remember we are not counsellors and we do not have the skills to counsel people about where they need to go or what they need to think; we can only listen, support and know when to refer to other professionals.

Emotional imbalances can be kept quite close to the surface in some people while in others they can be locked away exceptionally tightly. In the emotionally available people, the power of touch and empathetic listening can release things easily and is usually for the best. For those that have deep emotional reserves, release won't come easily and sometimes not at all. Occasionally it is important for that client's mental well-being that those emotions stay closed away as this is simply how they have learnt best to cope with their personal issues. If you have a client that your gut feeling tells you is not at all open or aware of their emotions, then do not push them into thinking about them. Whatever is right for your client will come naturally whenever it is the right time for it to do so.

We also need to recognise that as therapists we should do what is right for our own wellbeing too; you should always work within your comfort zone and experience, and anything that sits outside of it will not be right for you. The only person that can decide where your comfort zone lies is you.

Reflexology is an amazing therapy. We all know of clients who have benefited immensely from the balancing effects of therapeutic touch provided by a well-trained reflexologist. Some clients may need no more than reflexology touch to benefit; others may need reflexology and a listening ear. However, there may be those clients that are receptive to the concept where the additional dimension of the understanding of potential emotions can provide an extra level of support and release.

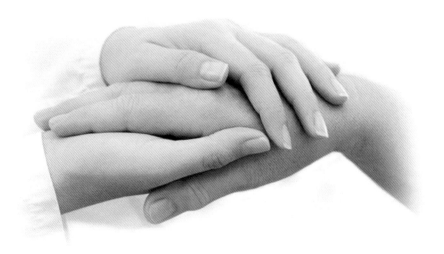

General introduction to emotions in the feet

There can be much to see on a pair of feet at first glance. Hard skin or any other form of difference can of course be due to imbalances in the reflexes due to practical reasons such as stance, gait, weight, infection and footwear, and these should be the first areas investigated.

Secondly, the hard skin could be due to protection of a physically related imbalance at that reflex point. Asking questions about the physical health may unearth issues from a long time ago that your client considers to be 'over, in the past, a long time ago' yet may still be present as an imbalanced reflex in the feet.

If none of these are relevant, then the potential for emotional imbalances comes to the fore. An awareness of how these show in any of the key emotional areas may help with unleashing a pent up or withheld emotion, allowing release.

Emotional imbalances may show in certain individuals as:

- Hard skin/callus represents an area of protection.
- Corns are similar to calluses and represent protecting a specific issue.
- Itching skin indicates irritation.
- Rough skin means going through a rough time.
- Damp skin can indicate anxiety but also could be a detox reaction.
- A verruca can be a deep rooted issue so bad that it is eating away at you.
- Athlete's foot represents someone getting under your skin, interfering, doubting, questioning your ideas and hindering your process (remember it needs treating physically too).
- Blister – someone is rubbing you up the wrong way and you're coming off worse!
- Dry skin indicates a need for more warmth, nurturing, or love.
- Peeling is about a fresh start or new beginning.
- Constant peeling indicates you think you dealt with the issue but it keeps coming back to haunt you.
- Oedema or swelling on the reflexes – when an emotion has been pent up for so long that there starts to be an emotional build up.
- The colour may indicate which emotion is involved.

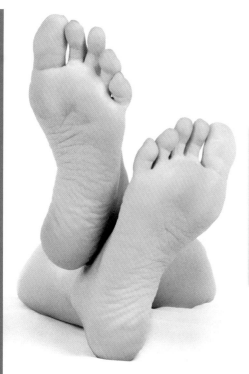

*Skin tone colours showing across a reflex:

Red – anger

Yellow – fed up

Blue – hurt

White – exhausted, drained or tired

Putting these together; a verucca on the lung reflex might represent a deep rooted issue in the emotional life. A red swelling on the heart reflex could represent anger about giving or receiving enough love, while a yellow area could be about being fed up with not receiving enough love. These concepts can then be gently introduced to your clients. Depending on how well you know them, you can be less - or more - forthright in your conversation. We have offered some areas for consideration and gentle discussion with the client, but don't feel you should use them all in one go. Gently add in the odd question and see if anything resonates with your client. If it does, then let them discuss it with you while you provide an empathic listening ear. Being listened to (and heard) can in itself be very healing.

Some reflexes are too small to have a separate, specific emotion attached. If you come across one of these then go with the prompts for the wider system.

Of course if your client doesn't have any awareness of issues in their emotional life, do not push your ideas onto them. Some people simply do not recognise emotions and that is how they get through their life. If this works for them, then that is how they need to be left; do not keep trying the emotional route if you meet with resistance.

There is also the issue of left and right foot reflexes – do these show different things? It is generally accepted that the right foot is past while the left foot is present. This can show in situations where you have a problem in a reflex that is on both feet but the imbalance only shows in one foot. This sometimes happens in the case of a chest infection, for example. It shows in the left foot reflex first (present) at one treatment, and then may pass to the right lung reflex in the next treatment (past). Subsequent treatments may not show any imbalances because the energy imbalance has left.

This situation can also happen with emotions – those long buried ones may appear in the right foot first, while those that are prompted by something in the present appear on the left. Of course, long buried emotions may also be re-ignited by something emotionally irritating in the present.

The right foot is also sometimes referred to as the male foot and the left as the female foot. This can relate to both male and female energy and also how we relate to men and women. If the past/ present issues do not appear to ring true then you can try the male/ female link. For example if the right foot is tense this may mean that there is a lack of male energy (yang) which is light, warm and active or that there has been issues or conflicts with a male e.g. father, brother or friend. If the left foot is tense, this can mean there is a lack of female energy (yin) which is dark, cool and restful, or there have been issues or conflicts with females e.g. mothers, sisters etc. You may find that for women with menstrual problems or in the process of becoming menopausal that the whole left foot may be more tender.

Another idea to consider if the reflexes are out of balance on one foot and not the other is that right foot reflexes are sometimes considered to be about processing, whilst those on the left foot can be about elimination (from a physical perspective rather than an emotional one).

Such instances may or may not occur in your client's feet; these examples are provided for your information and knowledge just in case you find it happens in one of your own treatments.

The Emotions in the Feet: A quick reference guide

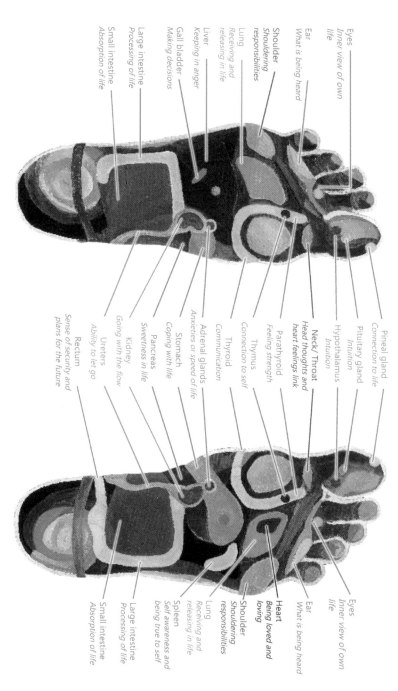

Plantar

Eyes
Inner view of own life

Inner view of own
life

Ear
What is being heard

Shoulder
Shouldering responsibilities

Lung
Receiving and releasing in life

Liver
Keeping in anger

Gall bladder
Making decisions

Large intestine
Processing of life

Small intestine
Absorption of life

Pineal gland
Connection to life

Pituitary gland
Intuition

Hypothalamus
Intuition

Neck/ Throat
Head thoughts and heart feelings link

Parathyroid
Feeling strength

Thymus
Connection to self

Thyroid
Communication

Adrenal glands
Anxieties or speed of life

Stomach
Coping with life

Pancreas
Sweetness in life

Kidney
Going with the flow

Ureters
Ability to let go

Rectum
Sense of security and plans for the future

Eyes
Inner view of own life

Ear
What is being heard

Heart
Being loved and loving

Shoulder
Shouldering responsibilities

Lung
Receiving and releasing in life

Spleen
Self awareness and being true to self

Large intestine
Processing of life

Small intestine
Absorption of life

Dorsal

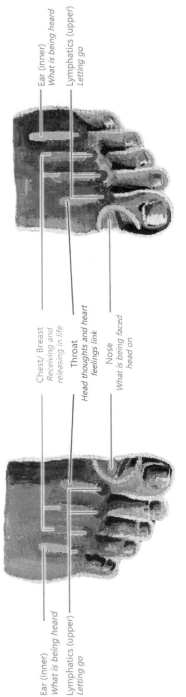

Ear (inner)
What is being heard

Lymphatics (upper)
Letting go

Chest/ Breast
Receiving and releasing in life

Throat
Head thoughts and heart feelings link

Nose
What is being faced head on

Ear (inner)
What is being heard

Lymphatics (upper)
Letting go

Medial

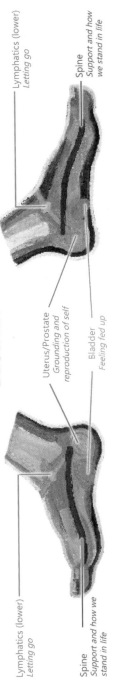

Lymphatics (lower)
Letting go

Spine
Support and how we stand in life

Uterus/Prostate
Grounding and reproduction of self

Bladder
Feeling fed up

Lymphatics (lower)
Letting go

Spine
Support and how we stand in life

Lateral

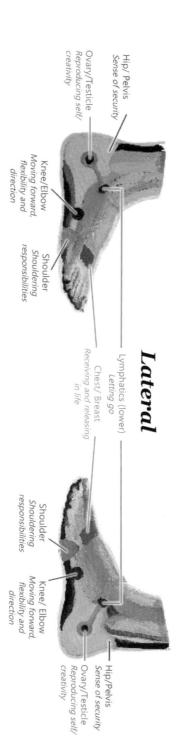

Hip/ Pelvis
Sense of security

Ovary/Testicle
Reproducing self/ creativity

Knee/Elbow
Moving forward, flexibility and direction

Shoulder
Shouldering responsibilities

Lymphatics (lower)
Letting go

Chest/ Breast
Receiving and releasing in life

Shoulder
Shouldering responsibilities

Knee/ Elbow
Moving forward, flexibility and direction

Hip/Pelvis
Sense of security

Ovary/Testicle
Reproducing self/ creativity

The Circulatory System

Introduction

The circulatory system consists of the fast cardiovascular system in addition to the slower lymphatic system. Together, these transport life giving components around the body; provide immunity to help fight infection and illness, and maintain homeostasis via the hormones. It takes amino acids, electrolytes and oxygen to where they are required and in return removes the waste products (including carbon dioxide) by passing them to the organs of excretion. Blood is an important carrier and there is approximately 4.7 to 5.7 litres of blood in each individual. A functioning immune system is provided by the white blood cells, while the red blood cells carry the oxygen.

Cardiovascular system

Introduction

The cardiovascular system is a closed system where the blood is enclosed in the vascular system throughout its journey.

There are two circulation loops:

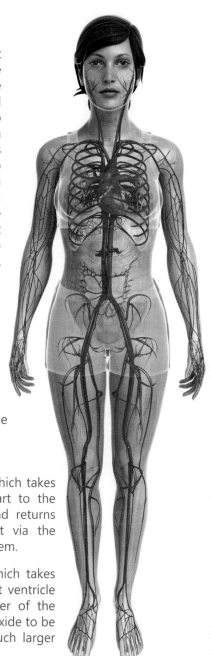

- the pulmonary loop (lung based) which takes deoxygenated blood from the heart to the lungs via the pulmonary artery and returns re-oxygenated blood to the heart via the pulmonary vein. A local yet vital system.

- the systemic loop (body based) which takes the oxygenated blood from the left ventricle via the aorta around the remainder of the body and picks up waste carbon dioxide to be released at the lungs. This is a much larger system as it takes in all of the body.

These systems are separated from each other by the heart.

Heart

Location in the body

The heart is slightly to the left of central in the upper torso.

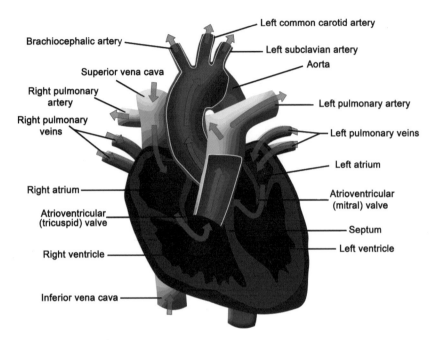

Left common carotid artery

Brachiocephalic artery

Left subclavian artery

Aorta

Superior vena cava

Right pulmonary artery

Left pulmonary artery

Right pulmonary veins

Left pulmonary veins

Left atrium

Right atrium

Atrioventricular (mitral) valve

Atrioventricular (tricuspid) valve

Septum

Left ventricle

Right ventricle

Inferior vena cava

Location in the feet

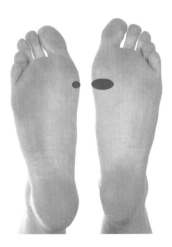

Pinch on the crease at the base of the ball of the foot. The heart reflex is more represented in the left foot than the right.

Location in the hands

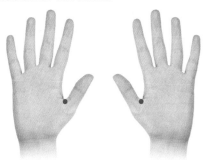

Pinch at the base of the thumb and first finger, the heart reflex is more represented in the left hand than the right.

Physiological action

The heart is a complex pump with four compartments. Two receive the deoxygenated blood and send it to the lungs and the other two receive the oxygenated blood and send it around the body. Each side has an atrium and a ventricle connected to each other by a major valve. The blood flows into the right atrium from the vena cave (at this point is it deoxygenated) and it passes via the valve into the right ventricle where it is pushed out to the lungs via the pulmonary artery. Here the haemoglobin molecules in the blood give up their bound carbon dioxide in exchange for the preferred oxygen molecules and return to the left atrium of heart via the pulmonary vein, passing again through a major valve. The oxygenated blood is squeezed out via the left ventricle through the aorta to the rest of the body. The oxygenated and deoxygenated sides of the heart do not mix.

The heart has its own circulation arising from the aorta, which provides nourishment to the heart muscle (myocardium). These are the coronary arteries and are the ones that are most likely to become damaged, causing angina or heart attacks.

Remember to state that reflexology is a sensitive therapy that can pick up current issues and past issues – it does not mean there are any major problems and may relate to a physical or an emotional imbalance in the body.

This is particularly important for the heart as you do not want clients to feel they have a physical problem with their heart. Always leave clients feeling reassured.

If the Heart reflex is out of balance, consider:

Physical prompts:

- Are they aware of any issues with their heart or circulation either currently or in the past?

- When they are feeling stressed, do they feel their heart racing?

- Do they get any aerobic exercise which allows the heart muscles to work efficiently? *Be aware this could be a sign of excessive exercise or too little.*

- Do they hunch over a computer? *This may restrict the flow of blood and energy through the heart.*

Arteries/ Arterioles/ Capillaries

Arteries are blood vessels that carry blood away from the heart, so they carry oxygenated blood (with the exception of the pulmonary and umbilical arteries). They have to take the high pressure strain of the heart pumping approximately 70 beats per minute and so consist of thick smooth muscle and elastin lined tubes, the composition of which alters depending on the role of the vessel. The main artery (the aorta) branches to become the systemic arteries supplying major organs; here they become smaller and smaller until they are called arterioles. These are involved in the regulation of blood pressure, having the ability to vary the contraction of the smooth muscle in their enclosing walls.

The arterioles feed the capillary beds where the exchange of gases and nutrients from the blood to the tissues takes place. Here the blood pressure drops as the blood travels though tiny tubes less than one blood cell wide, so the cells have to deform slightly to pass.

Capillary beds perform different actions depending where they are situated.

- In the lungs - carbon dioxide is exchanged for oxygen.

- In the tissues - oxygen, carbon dioxide, nutrients, and wastes are exchanged.

- In the kidneys - waste products are released to be eliminated from the body.

- In the intestine - nutrients are picked up, and waste products released.

Venules/ Veins/ Vena Cavae

After passing through the capillary beds, the blood cells are deoxygenated and carrying waste products. From here they flow into the venules, which are small, less muscular vessels that are very porous allowing for diffusion of fluid and cells. This is especially important around lymph nodes, where white blood cells encounter infections. Many venules join together to drain into one vein. Veins contain approximately 70% of the total blood volume, of which 25% is contained in the venules.

The walls of veins are composed of only thin layers of muscle as they are not required to function in a contractile manner and they have valves to prevent reverse blood flow. The return of the blood to the heart is assisted by the skeletal muscle pump, which is a collection of muscles required for standing and whenever they contract, they help the venous return to the heart. The blood flows through a valve and cannot flow back, while the contraction of the nearby muscle adds to the movement of the blood flow. The difference between veins and arteries is the direction of flow: veins towards the heart, arteries away from it - not whether they are carrying oxygenated or deoxygenated blood.

Location on the hands and feet

The circulatory system is extensive and present all over the body; therefore any effleurage or all over stroking of the hands and feet will be relaxing to the circulation.

Physical problems or illnesses to be aware of:

When thinking of the circulatory system, it is important to think of all the physical issues that might affect the whole system and check to see if there are any present now, or whether there have been any problems in this area in the past.

Examples might be:

Angina - a syndrome caused by a restriction of the blood supply to the heart. There are 2 types: stable and unstable. In stable angina, the symptoms are brought on by exercise, subside at rest, and usually develop gradually over time. In unstable angina, the symptoms develop rapidly and can persist at rest.

Arteriosclerosis - the thickening, hardening and loss of elasticity of the walls of arteries.

Atherosclerosis - a progressive condition in which the medium and large arteries become clogged by cholesterol and fatty substances. It is a type of arteriosclerosis.

Congenital Heart Disease - one or more defects of the heart that are present from birth. There are two main types – cyanotic and acyanotic. When the heart defect results in too little oxygen in the blood, it is called cyanotic heart disease. In acyanotic heart disease, there is sufficient oxygen in the blood but the defect in the heart prevents the blood from being circulated correctly.

Deep vein thrombosis (DVT) - formation of a blood clot within a deep lying vein, usually in the leg. Also called venous thrombosis.

Heart attack - sudden loss of blood supply to part of the heart muscle. The medical term for this is myocardial infarction and it is also commonly called a coronary.

Hypertension - persistent high blood pressure (in excess of 140/90mmHg) that may damage the arteries or heart.

Hypotension - lower than normal blood pressure.

Pulmonary Embolism (PE) - obstruction of the blood flow to the lungs by one or more blood clots.

Raynaud's Syndrome - sudden, intermittent narrowing of the arteries in the hands or, more rarely, the feet.

Thrombophlebitis (superficial) - inflammation of a vein, commonly a varicose vein, just below the surface of the skin that causes a blood clot. (Note: thrombus = blood clot, phlebitis = inflammation of a vein)

Varicose veins - Swollen and enlarged veins caused by the weakening of the valves that prevent the backflow of blood in the veins.

As there is not a specific reflex that would be out of balance, consider:

- Do they get cold feet and hands?
- Are they aware of any circulatory problems now or in the past?
- Have they had any physical problems with their heart?
- Do they have any areas of venous stagnation – blue or painful areas in the legs for example?
- Do they suffer from Raynaud's Syndrome – white or blue painful fingers when cold?

Emotional links: circulatory system

If physical issues are present, the emotional involvement may still be an important as part of the illness. If none of these are present, then it is even more important to consider emotional blocks.

Key area: all about love and being loved

The circulatory system is the flow of blood around the body, both oxygenated and deoxygenated. Blood is pumped by the heart. The theme of the heart is love. So blood is the chi (energy) or flow of love.

The heart is a 'love pump' and circulatory issues are to do with loving or not loving life and the ability to truly love and be loved.

Loving and being loved are two very different elements of life. Some people are very loving but find it hard to accept and receive love (as in receiving compliments, for example). Some people need to be loved but find it hard to truly and deeply love others. The ability to love and be loved is when great circulation can be most facilitated. The act of receiving a reflexology treatment is an example of being loved and loving the self - enough to get help and support.

If there is an issue with blood reaching the far extremities of the person's body and they are cold then this indicates that there is a potential belief that there is not enough love to go around; that they don't deserve love or that as they receive it, they give it straight back out.

Heart energy (love) in = Heart energy (love) straight out again.

The more the person loves and is loved (and when it's genuinely accepted and received), the better it is for heart energy and circulation in general. Love feeds the heart. Both giving and receiving in balance. Some people love others and do not take care of (or love) self. The better we get at loving ourselves, the better it is for everyone.

Emotionally, varicose veins are when there is blood (love) flowing and then running out of energy to get the blood back to heart centre to feed self again. The oxygen has been transported; however, there is a weakness in the return to self. Giving out or giving to others is okay, but not giving to self is difficult for the individual and could represent a weak system.

High blood pressure is when there is high pressure on things they love. High pressure and demands from and for loved ones / loved things and aspects of life they love. For example, when a man loves his family, his job, his car and playing football, it's a lot of outgoing love that becomes a pressure to manage and sustain.

Low blood pressure is when they have potentially given it (love) all out and have not received in equal quantities either due to lack of self-love, over-giving (love) or lack of loving being given/received. For example, a woman loves her family, her garden and taking the children to their hobbies. She gets exhausted in the process of giving out so much love and being in a situation where she perceives it's not always reciprocated in a balanced way.

Be aware as you listen, not to tell them how you think they should move forward, but instead ask useful questions to allow them to explore the ideas.

Please note: Exploring possible emotional reasons for reflexes that are out of balance has to be handled with great sensitivity, and can be presented purely as one school of thought. It may be that it is not suitable to share this information with your client, but it might help you understand why the reflex is imbalanced. You will need to use careful judgement as to whether to share this information.

If the Heart reflex is out of balance, consider issues relating to love:

Emotional prompts:

- What fills the client with love?
- What does the client love?
- Is the amount that they love equal to the amount that they are loved? Is one easier than the other for them?
- Is it safe to love and be loved? *Many have been deeply hurt and as a result fear loving and being loved due to past experiences including rejection and deep hurt.*
- Do they feel that they have enough love?
- If there is a line across the heart reflex - has the client experienced heartache or deep seated grief?

The Lymphatic System

Introduction

The lymphatic system is a series of blind ended tubes that travel all over the body. Throughout the network of lymph vessels there are small colonies of cells called lymph nodes that are a vital part of the immune response. There are gatherings of these lymph nodes in the groin, armpit (axilla), neck, abdomen and chest, which have a major role in the immune defence of the body. The lymph system drains into the circulatory system via two portals: the largest lymphatic vessel (the thoracic duct) passes into the left subclavian vein, and the smaller right lymphatic duct, which passes into the right subclavian and internal jugular veins. The right thorax, arm, head and neck drain into the right lymphatic duct, while the remaining three quarters of the body drains into the thoracic duct. This is where the slower lymphatic circulation joins the faster, pumped cardiovascular system. They are two halves of a whole circulatory system. At the lower end of the thoracic duct at the level of lumbar 1 and 2, there is also a dilated sac called the cisterna chyli. This is where lymph from the intestines - including the digested fats broken down to free amino acids (chyle) - is passed into the lymph system.

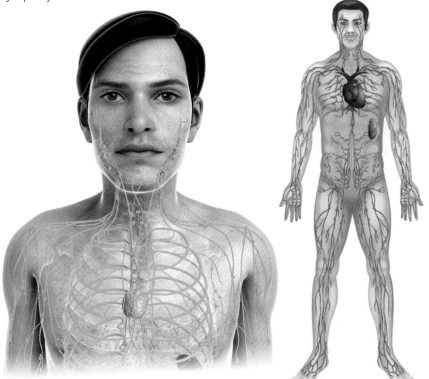

Location in the body

The lymphatic system runs throughout the body.

Location on the feet

Upper lymphatics

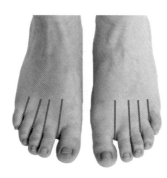

On the dorsal aspect of the feet thumb (or finger), walk between the metatarsal bones.

Lower lymphatics

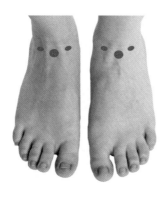

On the dorsal aspect of the feet, thumb (or finger) walk from ankle bone to ankle bone.

Location on the hands

Upper lymphatics

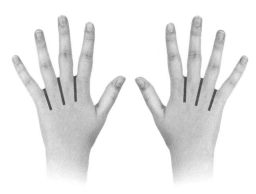

On the dorsal aspect of the hand, thumb (or finger) walk between the metacarpal bones.

Lower lympahatics

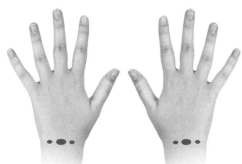

On the dorsal aspect of the hand, thumb (or finger) walk wrist bone to wrist bone.

Physiological action

The lymphatic system has three major roles:

- To remove waste products.
- To balance the body's fluid by draining and transporting the body's fluids back into the cardiovascular system.
- In immune defence, it is a part of the whole immune system, storing and moving lymphocytes.

About three litres of fluid is present at any one time in the lymph system, mainly in the interstitial spaces or the spaces between the cells. This fluid plays a crucial part of the removal of waste products from the metabolism of the cells.

The lymph fluid comes from the circulation, originating as plasma (the straw-coloured fluid that surrounds the blood cells). This then passes through the vascular wall into the spaces between the cells where it is then called interstitial fluid. Here it picks up waste products from the tissues and then passes through the walls of the lymph system, where it becomes lymph fluid. From here the lymph system moves the fluid by the action of external muscles, through a series of valves towards the heart. The fluid then re-enters the circulation at the subclavian vein or thoracic duct, where it becomes part of the circulatory system again. The waste products from between the cells are then filtered out via the kidneys to become urine.

Lymphatic tubes run very closely to the blood vessels but they differ in structure quite radically. Where the blood vessels have muscular walls and valves, the lymphatic tubes are very simple and not at all muscular. They have unidirectional valves but rely on the action of muscles around them for the movement of the lymph fluid.

The fact that the lymph system does not have its own muscular structure means it relies on the movement of the external muscles. When a person remains sedentary for long periods of time (especially under the pressure of an airline cabin, for example), the lymph fluid can find it hard to travel against gravity and it can pool in the ankles, causing swollen feet.

Throughout the network of lymph vessels there are small colonies of cells called lymph nodes that are a vital part of the immune response. There are gatherings of these lymph nodes in the groin, armpit, neck, abdomen and chest which have a major role in the immune defence of the body. These act both as filters and activation sites for an increased immune response. The lymph fluid flows through the lymph nodes bringing with it selections of foreign material, which may be from bacteria, viruses or damaged cells. This foreignness produces a reaction in the lymph node which, depending on the part of the immune system stimulated, may result in increased numbers of B cells, T cells or macrophages into the lymph and then into the circulation.

The spleen

Location in body

The spleen is a bean shaped organ that is in the left hand quadrant of the abdomen. An easy way to remember the anatomy of the spleen is the 1×3×5×7×9×11 rule. The spleen is 1" by 3" by 5", weighs approximately 7oz, and lies between the 9th and 11th ribs on the left hand side. It receives blood through both the gastric and splenic arteries, while the outgoing fluid (efferent lymph) exits into the lymphatic vessels.

Location on the feet:

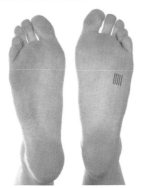

Left foot only - Thumb walk or knuckle down below the diaphragm line in Zones 4 to 5, to just above the waist line.

Location on the hands

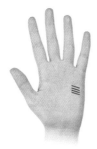

Left hand only - Thumb walk or knuckle down below the diaphragm line in Zones 4 to 5, to halfway down the palm.

Physiological action

The spleen has a similar structure to a lymph node, with clearly defined areas called red and white pulp.

The white pulp is very similar to the germinal centres of the lymph node; it is responsible for the synthesis of antibodies and is the centre of activity of the mononuclear phagocyte systems. As such, it is central to both humoral and cell mediated types of immunity; however, it is possible for the spleen to be surgically removed from the body, as most of its functions would be taken over by other organs. Nevertheless, it is common practice to prescribe long term antibiotics after a splenectomy to reduce the risk of bacterial infections.

The red pulp acts as a filter for the blood removing old red blood cells. The spleen recycles the iron recovered from the dead cells, which is then used in the production of new cells.

The spleen also holds the important role of retaining a large reserve of blood. This is particularly important in situations of haemorrhagic shock.

The thymus gland

Location in body

This is a small pinkish grey organ that sits in the middle of the chest above the heart. It is comparatively large at birth (about 5 cms in length) and increases in size until puberty, when it starts to atrophy with age. It is hardly visible as a separate organ in older age. The increase in sex hormones at puberty causes the reduction in size.

The thymus gland comprises two lobes, each of which are made up of follicles of 1 - 2cm, containing both a cortex and a medulla.

Location on the feet:

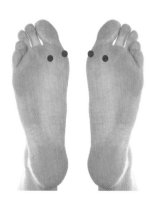

Squeeze either side of the big toe joint with your finger and thumb.

Location on the hands

Squeeze either side of the thumb joint with your finger and thumb.

Physiological action

The role of the thymus is mainly as part of the lymphatic system in younger life in educating and selecting T cells.

- The cortex (or outer area) contains mainly lymphocytes and a structural reticular network. Most of the body's T cell stock is built up in early life and passes through a selection process of gene rearrangement and positive selection.

- The medulla then completes the process by removing auto-reactive cells via negative selection through specialised cells called Hassel's corpuscles.

Physical problems or illnesses to be aware of:

When thinking of the lymphatic system, it is important to think of all the issues that might affect it and check to see if there are any present now, or whether there have been any problems in the past.

Some examples might be:

Infections - any type of infection, be it bacterial or viral, can have an effect on the lymphatic system. Even being close to someone with an infection can stimulate the immune system to react in protection mode.

Glandular fever - A viral infection causing swollen lymph nodes, a sore throat and fatigue. Also called infectious mononucleosis.

Haemorrhagic shock - rapid blood loss due to trauma, often resulting in a drop in blood pressure and tissue oxygenation.

HIV / AIDS - A long term infection which, if left untreated, results in reduced immunity to other infections.

Lymphadenopathy - enlarged lymph nodes usually due to a viral or bacterial infection.

Lymphoedema – localised accumulation of fluid in the lymphatic vessels causing swelling in the tissues. Post-operative scarring can also affect the flow of lymph, for example the occurrence of lymphoedema (swelling of the lymph system) is increased by surgery for breast cancer.

Lupus - Chronic autoimmune condition that causes inflammation in the body's tissues. There are 2 main types. The most common is systemic lupus erythematosus (SLE) which affects the whole body. Discoid lupus erythematosus only affects the skin.

Myesthenia Gravis - Literally means grave muscle weakness. It only affects voluntary muscles. This autoimmune disease can often be improved by the removal of the thymus.

Splenectomy – the removal of the spleen for various reasons results in an increased risk of infection by encapsulated bacteria such as the ones that cause bacterial meningitis due to the reduction in phagocyte activity.

Remember to state that reflexology is a sensitive therapy that can pick up current issues and past issues – it does not mean there are any major problems and may relate to a physical or an emotional imbalance in the body.

If the lymphatic system reflexes are out of balance, consider:

Physical prompts:

- Have they had any major infections in their life?
- Have they had any recent infections such as a cold or flu?
- Do they have any signs of 'killing off' infections such as a sore throat or sore glands?
- Do they have any swollen parts of their body?
- Have they had any major operations?
- Have they been in contact with anyone who has a bad infection? *Their body could be in protection mode.*

32

If these physical issues are present, the emotional involvement may still be an important as part of the illness. If none of these are present, then it is even more important to consider emotional blocks.

Key area: the ability to get rid of what no longer serves us.

The Lymphatic System is a little like looking at a map of the London underground where there are lots of stations (lymph nodes) and train lines (vessels) where all the passengers may be either just passing through or dropping off their waste products as they travel.

Exploring possible emotional reasons for reflexes that are out of balance has to be handled with great sensitivity, and it can be presented purely as one school of thought. It may be that it is not suitable to share this information with your client, but it might help you understand why the reflex is imbalanced. You will need to use careful judgement as to whether to share this information.

The lymphatic system is all about every kind of 'letting go' physically, emotionally, energetically or spiritually. Any fluid (lymph) that builds up represents withheld emotion (water equals emotion; e/motion equals energy in motion). Consider:

- What are they holding on to? (As opposed to having processed and let go of).

- Do they need to let go of something?

- Do they feel a bit stagnant?

As lymph is only moved due to movement of skeletal muscles, if there is no movement, the lymph (chi/energy) stagnates.

The area of the lymphatic fluid build-up will give more information of what the theme of their issue may be about. For example, swollen ankles equal withheld emotion and lack of flow to do with what a person stands for and how they stride out or forward.

Be aware as you listen, not to tell them how you think they should move forward, but instead ask useful questions to allow them to explore the ideas.

The Endocrine System

Introduction

The endocrine system is a group of glands that directly secrete hormones into the blood circulation. The hormones target a distant organ. It is a signalling system that has a slow initiation and a prolonged release and effect. The classic description of an endocrine organ is that it has high levels of blood supply, no ducts, and it has storage places for the hormone inside the organ, usually as vacuoles.

This is in contrast to the exocrine organs that have obvious ducts which release the product directly outside, examples of which are the sweat, salivary and mammary glands, and the liver.

Where there are glands that act by signalling in sequence through influence and feedback, it is known as an axis – the most well-known is the hypothalamus-pituitary-adrenal (HPA) axis.

The hypothalamus

Location in body

This is the nervous control system behind the endocrine system. It is a piece of neural tissue about the size of an almond, situated deep in the brain. It also anatomically sits on top of the pituitary.

Location on the feet

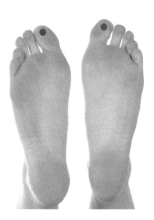

Find the whorl in the toe print, then place your fnger/ thumb just above it in the centre of the big toe. Push in and turn.

Location on the hands

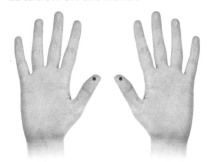

Find the whorl in the thumb print, then place your finger/ thumb just above it in the centre of the thumb. Push in and turn.

Physiological action of the hypothalamus

Its role is to make and secrete neuro-hormones or releasing factors, which have either a stimulatory or inhibitory effect on the pituitary gland. This provides the brain with a direct link to the endocrine system.

Remember to state that reflexology is a sensitive therapy that can pick up current issues and past issues – it does not mean there are any major problems and may relate to a physical or an emotional imbalance in the body.

If the hypothalamus reflex is out of balance, remember the primary function is to maintain homeostasis. The hypothalamus is involved in many necessary processes of the body including behavioural, autonomic and endocrine functions, such as metabolism, growth and development.

So consider if there are issues with:

- Physiological functions such as temperature regulation (may include hot flushes), thirst, hunger, sleep, fluid balance, blood pressure, mood, sex drive.

- Endocrine functions such as metabolism and growth and development in children.

- Physical and psychological effects of oxytocin – frequently referred to as the 'love hormone', oxytocin has an effect on bonding, stress, anxiety and depression, social skills, breastfeeding and childbirth etc.

Pituitary gland

Location in body

This is an endocrine gland the size of a pea that is linked to the hypothalamus by small tube (the pituitary stalk). This gland is very important and is protected by an outcrop of bone. It consists of two lobes with an indeterminate region between them:

Anterior lobe or adenohypophysis - fleshy and glandular tissue which regulates many physiological processes including stress, growth, reproduction and lactation.

Posterior lobe or neurohypophysis - neural tissue which releases anti-diuretic hormone and oxytocin.

In between the anterior and posterior lobes of the pituitary is an indistinct layer the intermediate layer which releases melanocyte stimulating hormones.

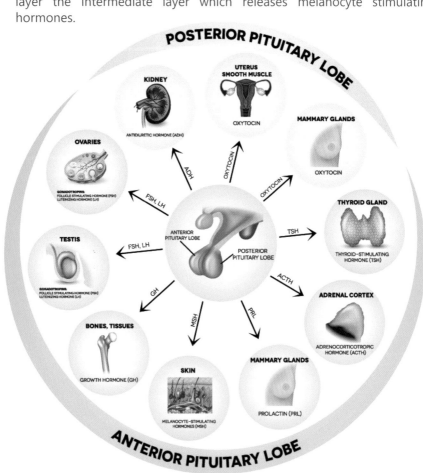

Location on the feet

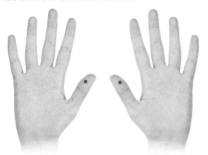

Place your index finger knuckle in the centre of the big toe. Look for the whorl in the toe print (between the first joint and the top); push in and turn.

Location on the hands

Place your index finger knuckle in the centre of the thumb. Look for the whorl in the thumb print (between the first joint and the top); push in and turn.

Physiological action of the pituitary gland

Anterior

- Prolactin – acts on the ovaries and the mammary glands to stimulate lactation, secretion of oestrogen and progesterone and also has other regulatory functions.

- Follicle stimulating hormone (FSH) – acts on the ovaries to cause the young small follicles to mature. Higher levels of oestrogen just before ovulation turn the production of FSH off.

- Luteinising hormone (LH) – acts on the ovaries to trigger the egg to release. Levels drop quickly afterwards.

- Adrenocorticotropic hormone (ACTH) – acts on the adrenal glands to stimulate aldosterone, the glucocorticoids and the androgens.

- Thyroid stimulating hormone (TSH) – affects the thyroid to stimulate production of thyroid hormones.

- Leptin - affects production of ACTH and TSH from their relevant cells.

- Growth hormone or somatotropin – acts on liver and fat tissue to promote growth and the metabolism of fat and carbohydrates.

- Beta endorphin – actions the opioid receptor to inhibit the perception of pain.

Posterior

- Antidiuretic hormone (ADH) – acts on the kidney to increase water retention and increase blood pressure by contracting the arterioles. It is also involved in male aggression.

- Oxytocin - affects the uterus and mammary glands to produce uterine contractions and lactation.

Intermediate

- Melanocyte stimulating hormones which acts on the receptors in the skin and hair to stimulate the release of melanin – increasing pigmentation in the skin.

Remember to state that reflexology is a sensitive therapy that can pick up current issues and past issues – it does not mean there are any major problems and may relate to a physical or an emotional imbalance in the body.

If the pituitary gland reflex is out of balance, consider:

Physical prompts:

- Have they been generally feeling 'out of sorts' hormone-wise?

- Are they very stressed?

N.B. High levels of stress can produce a negative feedback loop on the pituitary gland causing it to function less efficiently. The pituitary is also a very busy and important gland, so it is often slightly out of balance for no discernible reason.

Adrenal glands

Location in body

The adrenals are two glands that sit directly on top of both of the kidneys, which have a combined weight of about 7-10g in adults. They are under the action of hormones from the pituitary gland and produce hormones in response to stress.

They comprise an outer cortex and an inner medulla, which have different roles:

- Cortex - produces cortisol, aldosterone and androgens.

- Medulla - responsible for production of adrenalin (also known as epinephrine) and noradrenalin (also known as norepinephrine).

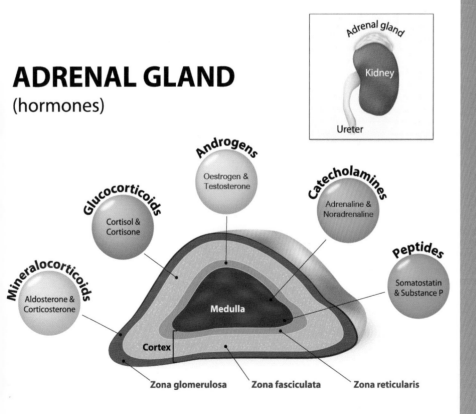

ADRENAL GLAND
(hormones)

Location on the feet

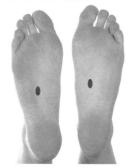

Press into zone two just above the kidneys on both feet. The left hand side adrenal is higher than the right hand side.

Location on the hands

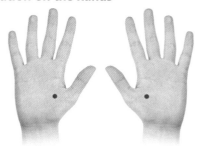

Pinch dorsal and palmar at the base of the webbing between the thumb and first finger.

Physiological action of the adrenal glands:

The hypothalamus signals the pituitary to make releasing factors that then act on the adrenal cortex to cause the production of:

- Aldosterone - increased reabsorption of calcium and increased secretion of potassium and hydrogen ions.

- Cortisol - mobilisation of fats, proteins and carbohydrates for increased energy supply to muscles. Also it enhances the activity of glucagon and the catecholamines (adrenalin and noradrenalin).

- Androgens - the best known is testosterone, responsible for the secondary male sex characteristics. In women, androgens initiate puberty, and have a life long role in the wellbeing of many organs and then become the route of oestrogen synthesis post-menopause.

The adrenal medulla receives messages from the sympathetic nervous system to synthesise the catecholamines - adrenalin and noradrenalin - as part of the 'fight or flight' response, resulting in an increase in heart rate, blood pressure, glucose release and greater blood flow to skeletal muscle in preparation for physical activity. They act through adreno-receptors throughout the body.

Remember to state that reflexology is a sensitive therapy that can pick up current issues and past issues – it does not mean there are any major problems and may relate to a physical or an emotional imbalance in the body.

If the adrenal gland reflex is out of balance, consider:

Physical prompts:

- Is the client very stressed at the moment or have they had periods of high stress in the past?

- Are they waking frequently in the night or finding it difficult to wake up in the morning?

- Do they feel their heart racing for no apparent reason?

N.B. rule out overuse of stimulants such as caffeine with the last point.

Pineal gland

Location in body

This is a pinecone shaped gland about the size of a grain of rice, set deep in the centre of the brain and attached to the thalamus. It is stimulated by light and inhibited by darkness and produces melatonin, a hormone derivative of serotonin. Tryptophan is a constituent of both molecules and is an essential amino acid (this means it is not synthesised in the body and so must be eaten) commonly found in protein rich foods such as meat, soya products, beans and nuts. It's also in chocolate and dairy products so perhaps this is why hot milk or chocolate is anecdotally supposed to aid sleep.

Location on the feet

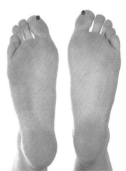

The pineal gland reflex can be worked on the top medial edge of the big toe. Some reflexologists place it on the top lateral edge of the big toe.

Location on the hands

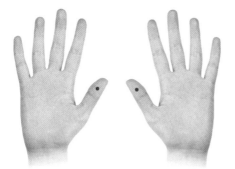

As the pineal sits behind the pituitary in the brain, working deeply on the pituitary (above) will also work the pineal.

Physiological action of the pineal gland:

The pineal gland produces melatonin - stimulated by light and inhibited by darkness, its circulating levels vary in a daily cycle which results in the biological entrainment (synchronisation to an external perceived rhythm) of circadian rhythms. It acts through specific receptors and has a role in the protection of DNA. It also regulates the production of leptin, the hormone that regulates fat storage in the body from fat cells.

Remember to state that reflexology is a sensitive therapy that can pick up current issues and past issues – it does not mean there are any major problems and may relate to a physical or an emotional imbalance in the body.

If the pineal gland reflex is out of balance, consider:

Physical prompts:

- Are they having trouble getting to sleep or staying asleep?

- Are they a frequent long-haul flyer?

- Do they have or have they had in the past any periods of jet lag?

- Do they do shift work?

N.B. you could mention the importance of getting light into the eyes for resetting the 'body clock'. Going out in the light every day is important , as is taking off glasses if they are worn, as they can block some of the critical wavelengths of light.

Thyroid gland

Location in body

One of the largest endocrine glands, the thyroid is situated in the neck just below the Adam's apple. It is composed of two lobes that produce a butterfly shape – each lobe is approximately 5cm x 3cm x 2cm. The thyroid is directly affected by the action of thyroid stimulating hormone (TSH) originating from the anterior pituitary, which is itself activated by thyrotropin releasing hormone from the hypothalamus.

Location on the feet

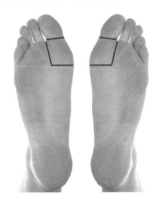

Work deeply at base of neck line for the thyroid and around the ball of foot for the thyroid helper area.

Location on the hands

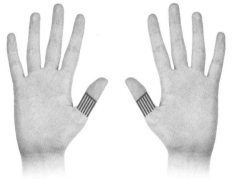

Work along the neckline and cover the base of the thumb to work the thyroid helper area.

Physiological action of the thyroid gland:

Three hormones are produced in the thyroid,

- Tri-iodothyronine (T3).
- Tetra-iodothyronine (T4), **better known as thyroxine.**

Both of these are formed from iodine and tyrosine molecules. They travel through the blood system to other organs such as the liver, kidney and spleen, and control how quickly energy is used. They are also involved in production of proteins, the use of the body's fat and glucose stores and the sensitivity of the body to other hormones. T3 and T4 increase the body's metabolic rate, which is how quickly cells use their stored energy. By controlling how much energy cells use, thyroid hormones also help to regulate body temperature. Heat is released when energy is used, thus increasing temperature.

- Calcitonin – this works together with parathyroid hormone to balance calcium and phosphate levels in the blood and bones.

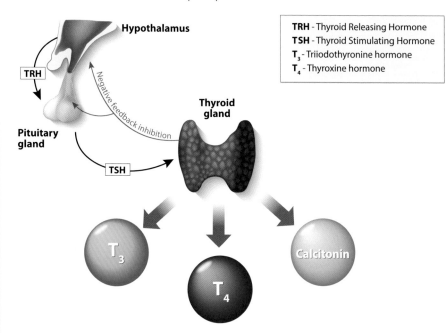

TRH - Thyroid Releasing Hormone	
TSH - Thyroid Stimulating Hormone	
T$_3$ - Triiodothyronine hormone	
T$_4$ - Thyroxine hormone	

Remember to state that reflexology is a sensitive therapy that can pick up current issues and past issues – it does not mean there are any major problems and may relate to a physical or an emotional imbalance in the body.

If the thyroid gland reflex is out of balance, consider:

Physical prompts:

- Do they often feel cold, have a lack of energy and put weight on easily?

- Do they feel hot, full of energy and lose weight at the drop of a hat?

N.B. these can be indications of hypo- or hyper- thyroid issues. If the client is experiencing these symptoms, you should advise your client to explain their symptoms to their GP and then tests may be offered.

Parathyroid glands

Location in body

These are 4 small flat ovoid discs resembling lentils on the back of the thyroid gland.

Location on the feet

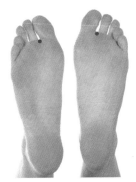

Work the lateral aspect of the big toe's second joint.

Location on the hands

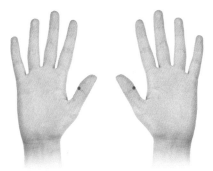

Work the lateral aspect of the thumb on the crease of the first joint.

Physiological action of the parathyroid glands

The parathyroid glands release parathyroid hormone, which together with calcitonin from the thyroid gland keeps the levels of calcium and phosphate in the blood and bones within tight control, through absorption and release when needed. This enables the nerves and muscles to work correctly.

Remember to state that reflexology is a sensitive therapy that can pick up current issues and past issues – it does not mean there are any major problems and may relate to a physical or an emotional imbalance in the body.

If the parathyroid gland reflex is out of balance, consider:

Physical prompts:

- Is the client prone to episodes of cramp?

- Has the client been diagnosed with osteoporosis?

- Is the client a menopausal woman, who is at higher risk?

Thymus gland

Location in body

This is a small pinkish grey organ that sits in the middle of the chest above the heart. It is comparatively large at birth at about 5cm in length, and increases in size until puberty. Once puberty is reached, it starts to atrophy with age and is hardly visible as a separate organ in older age. The increase in sex hormones at puberty causes the reduction in size.

It comprises of two lobes each of which are made up of follicles of 1- 2 cms, containing both a cortex and a medulla.

- The cortex or outer area contains mainly lymphocytes and a structural reticular network. Most of the body's T cell stock is built up in early life and passes through a selection process of gene rearrangement and positive selection in the thymus.

- The medulla then completes the process by removing auto-reactive cells via negative selection and specialised cells called Hassel's corpuscles.

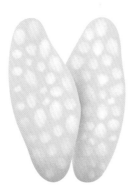

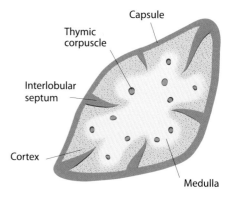

Location on the feet

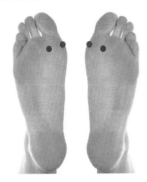

Squeeze either side of the big toe joint with your finger and thumb.

Location on the hands

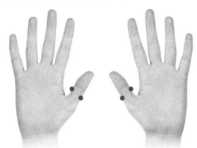

Squeeze either side of the thumb joint with your finger and thumb.

Physiological action of the thymus gland

The role of the thymus is mainly as part of the lymphatic system in younger life; however, it also has an endocrine function throughout life as it produces the hormone thymosin. This stimulates the maturation of T cells and is involved in the balance of the immune system.

Remember to state that reflexology is a sensitive therapy that can pick up current issues and past issues – it does not mean there are any major problems and may relate to a physical or an emotional imbalance in the body.

If the thymus gland reflex is out of balance, consider:

Physical prompts:

- Do they find it easy to get rid of any colds or infections?

- Do they have any indications that their immune system may be low?

Pancreas

Location in body

This is the largest of the endocrine organs, although there is also an exocrine function to a large proportion of the cells. It is a purplish fern shaped organ that lies behind the stomach and is 6 - 10cm long.

The endocrine function oversees the regulation of glucose metabolism and regulation, while the exocrine function helps with digestion.

Location on the feet

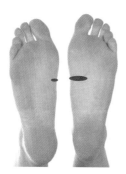

Thumb walk under the ball joint in Zone 1 on the right hand foot and Zones 1 and 2 of the left.

Location on the hands

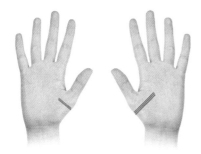

Thumb walk just below the base of the thumb on the right hand and across the base of the thumb and first finger on the left.

Physiological action of the pancreas:

The endocrine function of the pancreas arises from the Islets of Langerhans. These are dense areas of four cell types that are in direct contact with blood vessels. The cells are:

- Alpha cells - secrete glucagon, which increases blood sugar levels.
- Beta cells - secrete insulin, which decreases blood sugar levels.

- Delta cells - produces somatostatin which regulates the production of glucagon and insulin by the alpha and beta cells.

- PP cells - produce pancreatic polypeptide, which self-regulates pancreatic (both endocrine and exocrine) activities.

The exocrine function is the production of pancreatic fluid from the pancreatic cells into the pancreatic duct.

Remember to state that reflexology is a sensitive therapy that can pick up current issues and past issues – it does not mean there are any major problems and may relate to a physical or an emotional imbalance in the body.

If the pancreas reflex is out of balance, remember this could relate to endocrine or exocrine function. Consider:

Physical prompts:

- Do they get regular nausea, vomiting or had any weight loss?

- Are they aware if they have any problems with blood sugar levels?

- Has their diet changed, especially changes to the amount of sugar they eat?

- Do they ever feel like they could faint when they haven't eaten?

- Do they go to the loo more than usual?

* N.B. these could be symptoms of diabetes, so advise your client to take these symptoms to their GP where they might be offered further tests.

Ovaries

Location in body

These are the female part of the reproductive system and are located in the abdomen, one on either side. They are approximately 4cm x 3cm x 2cm in size. A female baby is born with all the eggs she will ever have, this is known as the ovarian reserve and as the female matures, so do the eggs. At puberty they begin to be released at a rate of approximately one per month, although it may vary with the individual. Every month, 20 or so follicles are stimulated and begin to mature to produce an egg, although usually only one will be released. Production of oestrogen, progesterone and testosterone in women comes from the ovaries.

Location on the feet

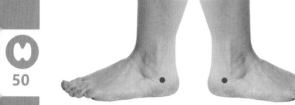

Press in the dip just above the heel bone in Zone 5 on the lateral ankle.

Location on the hands

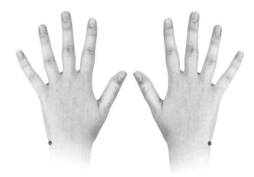

Press into the dip just in front of the wrist bone in Zone 5.

Physiological action of the ovaries:

In addition to their exocrine function of producing ova, the ovaries produce three hormones:

- Oestrogen - this is produced by the ovary and has a positive effect on the pituitary increasing production of lutinsing hormone (LH). Conversely, the same high levels reduce the production of Follicle Stimulating hormone (FSH). This turns off the egg maturation but turns on the egg release process.

- Progesterone – the ovary produces slowly increasing levels of this hormone over the second half of the cycle. Its job is to maintain the endometrium. If a fertilised embro implants, the endometrium remains thick and spongy ready for the placental growth. If there is no implantation, the progesterone concentration drops quickly, causing the endometrium to slough off. This results in a period.

- Testosterone – maintains bone density, muscle mass and energy levels and has an important role in women's sexual health.

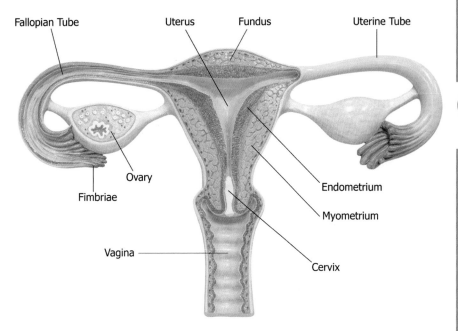

Fallopian Tube
Uterus
Fundus
Uterine Tube
Ovary
Fimbriae
Endometrium
Myometrium
Vagina
Cervix

Remember to state that reflexology is a sensitive therapy that can pick up current issues and past issues – it does not mean there are any major problems and may relate to a physical or an emotional imbalance in the body.

If the ovary reflexes are out of balance, consider:

Physical prompts:

- Do they have any problems that could be related to their periods?

Testes

Location in body

These are two egg shaped organs found in the scrotal sac. Their main functions are to produce sperm and androgens, including testosterone. The average testicular volume is 18cm³ (about 5cm x 2cm x 3cm). Release of the androgens is prompted by the action of gonadotropic hormones from the anterior pituitary.

Location on the feet

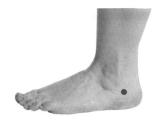

Press in the dip just above the heel bone in Zone 5 on the lateral ankle.

Location on the hands

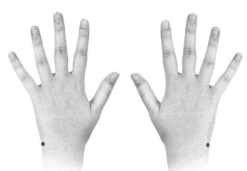

Press into the dip just in front of the wrist bone in Zone 5.

Physiological action:

In addition to their exocrine function of producing sperm, the testes produce one hormone:

- Testosterone - the release is caused by Luteinising Hormone (LH) from the anterior pituitary. It is required for the development of the male reproductive organs and provides the secondary sexual characteristics such as increased muscle, bone mass and body hair growth.

Both Follicle Stimulating Hormone (FSH) and testosterone are required for sperm production.

Adult males have 7-8 times the levels of testosterone compared to females but metabolise faster and so actually produce about 20 times more.

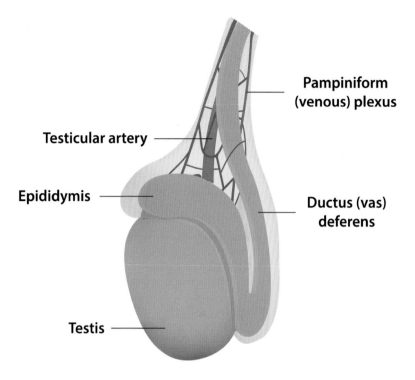

Pampiniform (venous) plexus

Testicular artery

Epididymis

Ductus (vas) deferens

Testis

Remember to state that reflexology is a sensitive therapy that can pick up current issues and past issues – it does not mean there are any major problems and may relate to a physical or an emotional imbalance in the body.

If the testes are out of balance, consider:

Physical prompts:

- Do they have any problems that could be related to their prostate?

- Do they have any problems urinating?

- Have they noticed any functional problems?

Physical problems or illnesses to be aware of:

When thinking of the endocrine system, it is important to think of all the issues that might affect the whole system and check to see if there are any present now, or whether there have been problems in the past.

Examples might be:

Stress - The reaction to stressors that causes a firing of the 'fight or flight' response through the hypothalamic pituitary adrenal axis (HPA) causing changes in the nervous and muscular systems.

54

Amenorrhoea - Absence of menstruation. There are 2 types – primary amenorrhoea, which is a failure to start menstruation, and secondary amenorrhoea, which is the absence of menstruation in a woman who has previously been menstruating.

Addison's disease - Disorder of the adrenal glands. Also known as primary adrenal insufficiency or hypo-adrenalism.

Cushing's syndrome - Hormonal disorder associated with high levels of steroid hormones.

Fibromyalgia - A chronic (long term) condition that causes pain all over the body. Also called fibromyalgia syndrome.

Diabetes Insipidus - Disorder caused by the body's inability to control its water balance. Not related to diabetes mellitus, although both conditions cause thirst and the excessive passing of urine.

Diabetes Mellitus (commonly called Diabetes) - Chronic condition caused by too much glucose in the blood. There are 2 types of diabetes mellitus - type 1 and type 2.

Dysmenorrhoea - Pain associated with menstruation.

Endometriosis - The presence of endometrial cells (the cells that line the interior wall of the uterus) in other parts of the body, such as the fallopian tubes, ovaries, bladder, bowel, vagina and rectum. These cells continue to be under the action of the normal cyclical hormones.

Infertility - the inability to conceive as a couple with a partner of normal fertility.

Fibroids - Non-cancerous tumours that grow slowly within the muscular wall of the uterus or around the uterus.

Hyperthryroidism - Overproduction of thyroid hormones. Also called thyrotoxicosis. It is one of the most common hormonal disorders.

Hypothyroidism - A low level of thyroid hormones in the blood.

Impotence (erectile dysfunction) - Inability to achieve or sustain an erection.

Insomnia - Regular inability to fall asleep or stay asleep.

Menorrhagia - Heavier than normal bleeding during menstruation.

Polycystic Ovary Syndrome (PCOS), also known as polycystic ovaries - Multiple small, fluid-filled cysts on the ovaries. Those with the syndrome will also have at least two of the following symptoms: irregular periods, high levels of androgens (which can cause weight gain, acne, depression and hirsutism) and polycystic ovaries.

Emotional links: Endocrine System

If these physical issues are present, the emotional involvement may still be important as part of the illness. If none of these are present then it is even more important to consider emotional blocks.

Key area: in general, the endocrine system relates to messages being sent and received.

If communication is hard, then it is hard for the messages to be received. If the person is living on red alert, the endocrine system will also be in a state of red alert, and there may be too many messages and alerts being activated and being processed. Their whole system can be overwhelmed, leaving the endocrine system functioning in a chaotic fashion. The endocrine system goes awry when there is too much input. Ideally, the endocrine system works in balance and harmony.

Be aware as you listen not to tell them how you think they should move forward, but instead ask useful questions to allow them to explore the ideas.

Exploring possible emotional reasons for reflexes that are out of balance has to be handled with great sensitivity, and can be presented purely as one school of thought. It may be that it is not suitable to share this information with your client, but it might help you understand why the reflex is imbalanced. You will need to use careful judgement as to whether to share this information.

The pituitary gland and hypothalamus: *These are all about our sixth sense. They are the houses of intuition or inner knowing. They are our internal radar and keep us connected to our intuition. When the pituitary and hypothalamus are working well and in balance, we find it easier to be connected to all of our senses and our intuition.*

- How is the client's intuition functioning at the moment? Are they trying to avoid it?

The pineal gland: *Atrophies over time and relates to keeping connection with the bigger picture. It is our connection to our "meaning of life."*

- Are they feeling disconnected from the world at the moment?

The thyroid gland: *The thyroid is the centre of our communication. It's our verbal and non-verbal, internal and external communication. It is the words (and tone) that we speak out into the world and the words (and tone) that we speak in our own heads - both the actual words and the body language, expressions and ways of living. Thyroid energy is all about communication in every possible way. Taking the communication link further, the thyroid reflex also indicates the emotional area to reflect self-esteem issues:*

- How is their self-esteem at the moment?

- What one thing specifically could they do today to boost their self-esteem?

If the thyroid is overactive, it's an indication that there is too much going on. If it is underactive then stagnation may be the cause. Not knowing and not being able to communicate themselves as they are, can cause stagnation and underactivity.

- Are they having problems communicating with someone in particular?

The parathyroid: *This is related to feeling strong.*

- Are they feeling that their strength is being sapped by something?

- Do they need to conserve their strength?

The thymus gland: *This is the centre of our loving connection to self and our body. The centre of the immune system is directly connected to our love of self.*

- Are they finding it hard to love themselves at the moment?

The pancreas: *This represents the processing of life and relates to how sweet it is – or not. Enzymes that the pancreas produces aid digestion and so this relates to the ability of the person to be able to break life down into small parcels/particles.*

Sometimes life is not sweet or the sweetness is lost. Looking at the small parts of life can make it easier to find the sweet things (nice things or small aspects of life that are okay). An imbalance in the pancreas which leads to more challenges with blood sugar levels can be caused by someone receiving a shock of significant proportion.

Shock can impact the function of the pancreas and the physical knock-on effects can be picked up within two years of the shock occurring.

The pancreas relates to confidence and creativity. Shock can negatively impact these. The resolution is to take tiny steps forward to increase creativity and confidence. With an increase of both of these, the person will have more energy, strength and ability to cope with any further life shocks. Being able to cope keeps the sweetness of life. Creatively keeping and re-finding or reconnecting with sweet moments is very empowering to anything pancreatic.

- In terms of what they are doing or what is being done, how can the client bring the sweetness back to what they are doing?

- How are they feeling about what they are doing or what is being done?

The adrenal glands: *Coping with life and life shocks, fears and anxiety. The adrenals are also associated with the pace of life; to speed, a speedy life and being able to respond immediately. If the adrenals are over working, the person may be living a life that is moving too fast.*

The adrenal gland/kidney reflexes are also located on the horizontal zone connected to doing energy and working life issues.

- Is the client very competitive? Even perhaps against themselves?

- How are things at work for them?

- What is it that they are doing or that is being done that is causing them stress?

- Are they doing too many things rather than focusing on just one?

- Can they swap activity to inactivity – busy head (thoughts) to calm thoughts, highly charged to very chilled?

The ovaries/testes: *Reproducing self. Do they want to replicate themselves? Is their life something they would like to replicate? It's about passing something forward for humanity to benefit by. If someone is unhappy with who they are and does not wish to replicate that or pass it forward, they are more likely to experience endocrine issues relating to the reproductive areas and this can be eased when someone finds more peace, love and acceptance for themselves and 'who vs. how' they are.*

Issues around the endocrine system may also be about creativity –

- Are they accessing their creative side enough?

- If they could create anything, what would they like to create?

- Are they unhappy about who they are?

The uterus area is representative of expansion and space, so you could consider:

- Are they planning a period of expansion?

- Do they have enough space to grow? (their family for example?)

- If fertility related, do they have enough room in their life for a(nother) baby?

The Excretory System

Introduction

Once the body has gained everything it needs from the food and drink it consumes and the various bodily processes have taken place, it is left with waste products which need to be excreted (removed) from the body in order to prevent damage and maintain homeostasis.

Waste is excreted from the body via the following substances:

- urine (involving the kidneys, ureter tubes and bladder).
- faeces (involving the large intestine, rectum and anus).
- expelled breath (involving the lungs).
- sweat (involving the skin, especially apocrine and eccrine glands).

The organs of excretion covered in this section include the kidneys, ureter tubes and bladder, which are all involved with the production and excretion of urine. Whilst our full excretory system does also comprise the large intestine, liver, skin and lungs, these components are all covered elsewhere in this book.

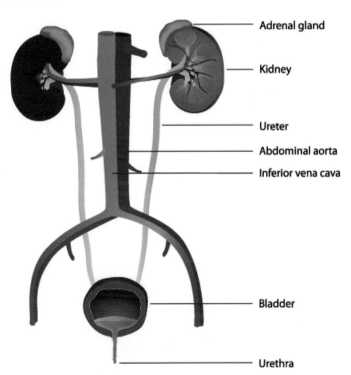

Adrenal gland

Kidney

Ureter

Abdominal aorta

Inferior vena cava

Bladder

Urethra

The Kidneys

Location in body

The kidneys are a pair of bean-shaped organs, each of which is about the size of a fist. They are situated in an asymmetrical way, with the right kidney being slightly lower down and more lateral than the left. They reside at the upper posterior part of the abdomen, with the left kidney being roughly level with vertebrae T11 through to L3. They sit one on each side of the body, either side of the spine.

Location on the feet

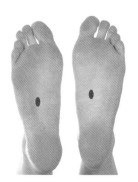

Push in and rotate just underneath and to the medial side of the solar plexus reflex. The left kidney is higher than the right kidney.

Location on the hands

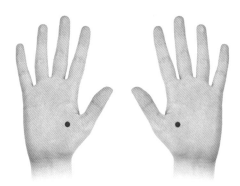

Pinch the dorsal and palmar reflexes at the base of the webbing between the thumb and first finger.

Physiological action of the kidneys

These regulate the volume of blood by removing excess water, salts and urea. 'Dirty' blood enters the kidneys and the waste is filtered out. 'Clean' blood re-enters the circulatory system whilst the waste (called urine) passes into the ureter tubes and onwards to the bladder.

Physical problems or illnesses to be aware of:

When thinking of the kidneys, it is important to think of all the issues that might affect them and check to see if there are any present now, or if there have been problems in this area in the past.

Examples might be:

Glomerulonephritis - the inflammation of the glomeruli (the filtering units) in the kidneys, which is characterised by blood and protein being passed in the urine.

Hydronephrosis - one or both kidneys stretching or swelling, commonly caused by a blockage somewhere in the urinary system.

Kidney stones, also known as nephrolithiasis - crystalline deposits that build up in one or both kidneys.

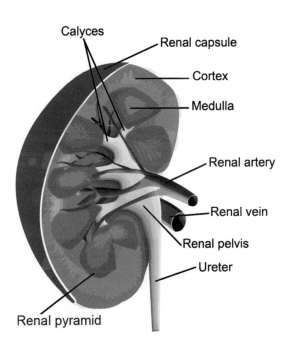

Kidney (Renal) failure - the loss of kidney function. This can be either acute (short term) or chronic (long term).

Pyelonephritis - a kidney infection which results in the swelling of one or both kidneys, which is usually caused by bacteria which have been transferred from the anus to the urethra, and which have then travelled upwards through the urinary system to the kidney.

Remember to state that reflexology is a sensitive therapy that can pick up current issues and past issues – it does not mean there are any major problems and may relate to a physical or an emotional imbalance in the body.

If the kidneys are out of balance, consider:

Physical prompts:

- Do they have or have they had any problems with their kidneys?

- Do they have or have they had any pain in their back around the level of their waist?

- Do they have or have they had any problems urinating?

- How has their water intake been recently?

- Have they noticed if their urine has changed in colour recently e.g. darker than normal?

- Have they been sweating more than usual? Has it been hot, have they been doing a lot of exercise or having hot sweats? All of these can mean that water is being lost through the skin, concentrating the waste products.

The ureter tubes

Location in body

The ureter tubes connect the kidneys in the upper posterior of the abdomen to the bladder in the medial lower abdomen. They are approximately 12 inches long.

Location on the feet

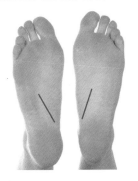

Thumb walk from the bladder to the kidney and then down from kidney to bladder to flush.

Location on the hands

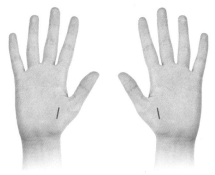

Thumb walk from the kidney reflex down to bladder point located in the centre of the muscle at base of thumb.

Physiological action of the ureter tubes

The ureter tubes transport waste fluid (urine) from the kidneys to the bladder.

Physical problems or illnesses to be aware of:

When thinking of the ureter tubes, it is important to think of all the problems that might affect them and check to see if there are any present now, or whether there have been any issues in the past.

An example would be:

Ureteral obstructions - blockages in one or both of the ureters.

Urinary tract infections - bacterial infections of the urinary tract that can spread upwards from the bladder through the ureters towards the kidneys.

Remember to state that reflexology is a sensitive therapy that can pick up current issues and past issues – it does not mean there are any major problems and may relate to a physical or an emotional imbalance in the body.

If the ureter tubes are out of balance, consider:

Physical prompts:

- Do they or have they had any problems urinating/passing water?
- How has their water intake been recently?
- Have they noticed if their urine has changed in colour recently e.g. darker than normal, as this may irritate the ureter tubes?
- Have they been sweating more than usual? Has it been hot, have they been doing a lot of exercise or having hot sweats? All of these can mean that water is being lost through the skin concentrating the waste products.

The bladder

Location in body

The bladder is a muscular sac in the medial part of the pelvis, situated just above and behind the pelvic bone.

Location on the feet

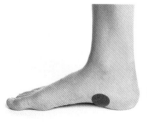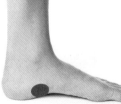

Push in and rotate on the bottom of the medial part of the foot (just in front of the ankle line).

Location on the hands

Push in and rotate in the middle of the muscle at the base of the thumb.

Physiological action of the bladder

Once in the bladder, the urine is stored until the body releases it via the urethra. Urination (or micturition) involves the contraction of the muscular walls of the bladder to push the urine out.

Physical problems or illnesses to be aware of:

When thinking of the bladder, it is important to think of all the issues that might affect it and check to see if there are any present now, or whether there have been any problems in the past.

Some examples might be:

Bladder stones - small mineral deposits that form in the bladder, which are normally caused by urine remaining in the bladder too long. These are more common in men than in women, and more common in those over the age of 45.

Cystitis - the inflammation of the bladder, normally caused by a bacterial infection.

Urinary incontinence - the involuntary release of urine, which can be a chronic (long-lasting) condition.

Urinary retention - where urine does not evacuate the bladder normally, due to either a blockage of the urethra or suppressed bladder muscle activity.

Remember to state that reflexology is a sensitive therapy that can pick up current issues and past issues - it does not mean there are any major problems and may relate to a physical or an emotional imbalance in the body.

If the bladder reflex is out of balance, consider:

Physical prompts:

- Do they have or have they had any problems with their bladder such as infections?

- Have they noticed if they are urinating/ passing water more often?

   If Yes: Does it hurt, feel like it's burning or feel itchy when they urinate, or do they feel like they don't empty their bladder fully? If these symptom persist for more than a few days then the client should arrange to see their GP to discuss their symptoms, as it may be a sign of an infection.

- Have they noticed if their urine has changed in colour recently e.g. darker than normal?

- How is their water intake?

- Have they been sweating more than usual - has it been hot, have they been doing a lot of exercise or having hot sweats? All of these can mean that water is being lost through the skin, concentrating the waste products.

The urethra

Location in body

The urethra is a tube that joins the bladder to the exterior of the body. The length and action of the tube differs in males and females.

Location on the feet:

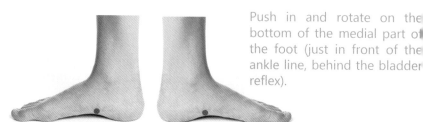

Push in and rotate on the bottom of the medial part of the foot (just in front of the ankle line, behind the bladder reflex).

66

Location on the hands

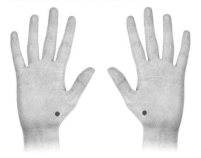

Push in and rotate in the middle of the muscle at the base of the thumb, just above the wrist.

Physiological action of the urethra

In women, the urethra solely conveys urine from the bladder to the exterior of the body.

In men, the urethra conveys urine from the bladder to the exterior of the body during urination, and semen from the testes and prostate gland to the exterior of the body during ejaculation.

Physical problems or illnesses to be aware of:

When thinking of the urethra, it is important to think of all the issues that might affect it and check to see if there are any present now, or whether there have been any problems in the past.

Non-specific urethritis - the inflammation of the urethra when it is not caused by gonorrhoea.

A urinary tract obstuction - a blockage anywhere in the urinary tract, including the urethra.

Urinary tract infections - bacterial infections of the urinary tract that can spread upwards from the bladder through the ureters towards the kidneys.

Remember to state that reflexology is a sensitive therapy that can pick up current issues and past issues – it does not mean there are any major problems and may relate to a physical or an emotional imbalance in the body.

If the urethra reflex is out of balance, consider:

Physical prompts:

- Does it hurt them, feel like it's burning or feel itchy when they urinate?

- Is there a discharge from the urethra?

- Do they have any pain in their lower pelvic region?

- Do they find they have difficulty urinating?

If these symptoms persist then the client should arrange to see their GP to discuss their symptoms, as it may be a sign of an infection or blockage.

Emotional links: Excretory system

If these physical are present, the emotional involvement may still be important as part of the illness. If none of these are present then it is even more important to consider emotional blocks.

Key area: support impacting on family or private life.

Be aware as you listen, not to tell them how you think they should move forward, but instead ask useful questions to allow them to explore the ideas.

Exploring possible emotional reasons for reflexes that are out of balance has to be handled with great sensitivity, and it can be presented purely as one school of thought. It may be that it is not suitable to share this information with your client, but it might help you understand why the reflex is imbalanced. You will need to use careful judgement as to whether to share this information.

The kidney: *represents 'going with the flow' of life. It also represents the house of fear because if you are frightened then it is difficult to 'go with the flow'. Its about learning to go with YOUR flow.*

- Are they fearful of something in their life?

- Are they fighting against going with the flow?

- Do they sometimes feel that they are 'swimming upstream' against issues?

An alternative view of this is that it represents 'the way you are thinking about how you are feeling is impacting on what you are doing or what is being done'.

- How are they feeling about what they are doing?

The kidney can also represent crying inside or unshed tears.

- Do they need to have a good cry about something?

The ureter: *related to the ability (or inability) to let let go.*

- Are they having issues with the letting go of some thought or emotion?
- Is there something in their life that they need to let go of?

The bladder: *relates to everything about being truly fed up – in other words – 'peed off'. When someone has an issue with their bladder, it is very often at a time when something has made them feel this way.*

- Have they been feeling fed up or peed off with someone or something recently?

It's also about holding onto things and being unable to let go or letting go in an extreme fashion. Bladder incontinence is when the general pressure of life is causing someone to be peed off (fed up) and something (the bladder) gives under pressure.

Bladder retention problems are when someone is trying to hang onto their flow of life, when life does not feel free-flowing. Urine is about flow – too fast, lack of, or painful.

- Are they feeling as though their life has stagnated?
- Is their life moving too fast?

The urethra: *spans over two emotional areas: those of family and work.*

a) The way they are thinking about how they are feeling impacting on what they are doing or what is being done.

b) The way they are thinking about their self-esteem or core beliefs and ideas is impacting on their private life.

- How are they feeling about what is being done?
- What's happening at work?
- Is their self-esteem impacting on how they relate to others?
- How are things between them and their family or partner?

The Digestive System

Introduction

The body needs to gain energy and nutrients from the food we eat. For this to happen, the body needs to break down the food we ingest into the smallest chemical components. This means it can then be absorbed into the blood stream by the small intestines and carried to every cell in the body for energy, growth, repair and general function. This process of breaking down foods is known as digestion.

The digestive system is responsible for:

- ingestion of food.
- mechanical and chemical digestion.
- absorption of nutrients and water.
- elimination of waste products.

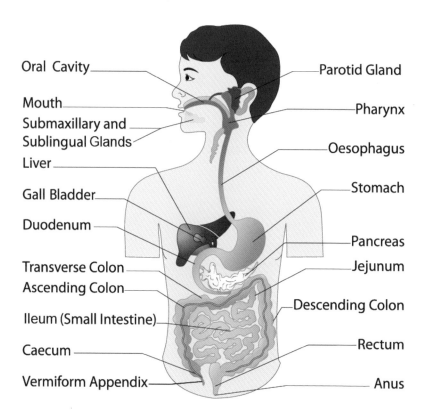

Oral Cavity — Parotid Gland
Mouth — Pharynx
Submaxillary and Sublingual Glands
Liver — Oesophagus
Gall Bladder — Stomach
Duodenum — Pancreas
Transverse Colon — Jejunum
Ascending Colon — Descending Colon
Ileum (Small Intestine) — Rectum
Caecum
Vermiform Appendix — Anus

The mouth

Location in body

The mouth, or oral cavity, is considered to be the start of the digestive tract, although the process of digestion actually starts before this; the smell of food stimulates the salivary glands to produce saliva, 'making our mouth water'.

Location on the feet

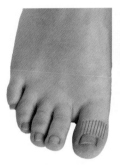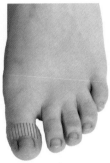

Use 2 or 3 fingers to walk down the dorsal aspect of the big toes from the base of the nail to the first joint.

Location on the hands

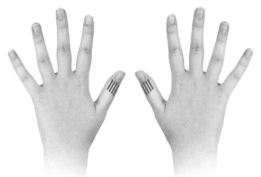

Use 2 or 3 fingers to walk down the dorsal aspect of the thumb from the base of the nail to the first crease.

Physiological action of the mouth

There are two types of digestion that occur in the mouth. Firstly, mechanical digestion takes place: the teeth grind the food and break it down (known as mastication) in preparation for swallowing and to prevent choking. Breaking the food down also creates a larger surface area which will allow enzymes to work more effectively for the second type of digestion: chemical digestion.

The mouth produces saliva from the salivary glands. This is 99.5% water, which helps to moisten the food to make swallowing easier. The salivary glands also produce the enzymes which are essential for starting the chemical digestion of foods:

- Amylase (produced by the parotid glands located at the back of the jaw) which breaks down carbohydrates.

- Protease (produced by the sub-mandibular glands located under the floor of the mouth) which begins protein digestion.

- Lipase (produced by the sublingual glands under the tongue) for fat digestion.

Saliva production is under the control of the autonomic nervous system (ANS). In response to the smell and/or taste of food, the ANS increases the blood flow through these glands which results in an increase in the production of saliva.

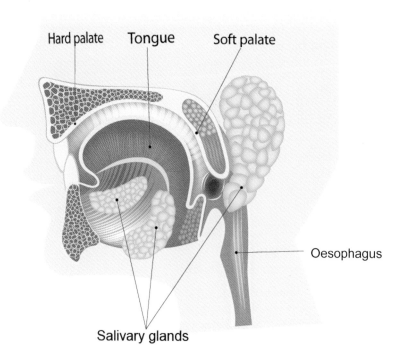

Hard palate   Tongue   Soft palate

Oesophagus

Salivary glands

Physical problems or illnesses to be aware of:

When thinking of the mouth, it is important to think of all the issues that might affect it and check to see if there are any present now, or whether there have been any problems in the past.

Dry mouth (also known as Xerostomia) results from reduced or absent saliva flow. It can be a symptom of various medical conditions, a side effect of radiotherapy to the head and neck, or a side effect of a wide variety of medication including many anti-depressants.

Gum disease is often a result of poor oral hygiene or lack of teeth brushing - it can lead to inflammation in the gum and eventually teeth can become loose and may fall out.

Mouth ulcers are painful round or oval sores that form in the mouth or on the lips. Mouth ulcers are extremely common and usually result from injury - e.g. biting the cheek. If they recur or are difficult to clear it can be a sign of other issues such as anaemia, fungal/bacterial/viral infection, or an iron or Vitamin B12 deficiency.

Remember to state that reflexology is a sensitive therapy that can pick up current issues and past issues – it does not mean there are any major problems and may relate to a physical or an emotional imbalance in the body.

If the mouth reflex is out of balance, think about this reflex area also covering jaw, teeth and throat. Consider:

Physical prompts:

- Do they have any current pain in their mouth, jaw, throat or teeth?
- Are they prone to any conditions or infections in their mouth, jaw, throat or teeth?
- Do they hold tension in their jaw when they are stressed?
- Do they suffer with a dry mouth – perhaps when they are stressed?
- Are they aware if they grind their teeth at night?
- If the jaw is out of balance, see if the client has had a hip problem. The two can be linked in reflexology theory.

Stomach

Location in the body

The stomach is a muscular, sac-like organ located in the left side of the upper abdomen below the diaphragm line. It is about 15cm wide and 30cm long; the size varies in different people and before and after meals as it can hold about 1L of food.

Location on the feet

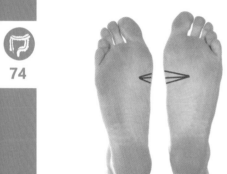

Walk from the medial edge of the foot, below the diaphragm line, across towards solar plexus. The stomach is primarily found on the left foot.

Location on the hands

The stomach reflex has two common placements:

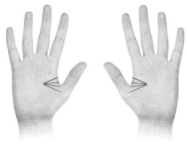

1. The webbing at the base of the thumb. Place your thumb at the base of the 'V' and walk a line towards the base of the thumb, draw back to the base of the 'V' and continue to walk in lines to cover the whole area.

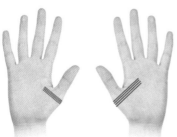

2. Positioned below the diaphragm line, largely on the left hand. Thumb walk across the area.

Physiological action of the stomach

As food enters into the stomach through the cardiac sphincter, this closes so the food remains in a closed sac for the next stage of chemical digestion. The stomach has several layers including the mucosa, which has glands that secrete hydrochloric acid and other glands that produce enzymes which work with the acid to break down the food. The muscular layer of the stomach contracts and relaxes to mix the food, ensuring that the acid and enzymes can get to work on all the food to produce a liquid called chyme. Small amounts of nutrients are absorbed by the mucosal layer of the stomach and the chyme then passes through the pyloric sphincter (a ring of muscle that acts as a valve) into the duodenum (the first part of the small intestines).

Physical problems or illnesses to be aware of:

When thinking of the stomach, it is important to think of all the issues that might affect it and check to see if there are any present now, or whether there have been any problems in the past.

Gastritis - inflammation of the lining of the stomach, which has many possible causes. Common causes of gastritis are excessive alcohol consumption or prolonged use of non-steroidal anti-inflammatory drugs (also known as NSAIDs) such as Aspirin or Ibuprofen.

Gastroenteritis - Inflammation of the lining of the stomach and intestines. Usually caused by either a viral infection (e.g. norovirus) or a bacterial infection (e.g. E.coli and salmonella). Bacterial infections are often picked up from contaminated food or water, and there is an increased risk of this when travelling abroad. Most forms of gastroenteritis are highly infectious and are passed from faeces to mouth via the hands when hygiene is poor.

Hiatus hernia - The protrusion of a portion of the stomach through the diaphragm. The general term "hernia" is used to describe the protrusion of a part of an organ through a weakened muscle. "Hiatus" is the opening in the diaphragm through which the oesophagus passes. The hiatus is the weakened area through which the stomach protrudes in a hiatus hernia.

Peptic ulcers - An open sore on the lining of the stomach (gastric ulcer) or on the lining of the first part of the small intestine (duodenal ulcer). The majority of peptic ulcers are due to an infection by the Helicobacter pylori bacteria. These bacteria damage the protective mucus lining of the stomach and small intestine, leaving the underlying tissue subject to erosion by the acidic digestive juices, allowing an open sore to form. Peptic ulcers can also be caused by the long term use of some drugs such as Aspirin and Ibuprofen, which damage the stomach lining. Risk factors include family history, smoking, and alcohol consumption. Stress may worsen the symptoms.

Pernicious anaemia - Anaemia is the term used to describe disorders in which the haemoglobin in the red blood cells is deficient or abnormal. Pernicious anaemia is an autoimmune disease that affects the stomach, preventing the absorption of vitamin B12. Vitamin B12 is one of the necessary components required to produce healthy red blood cells.

Remember to state that reflexology is a sensitive therapy that can pick up current issues and past issues – it does not mean there are any major problems and may relate to a physical or an emotional imbalance in the body.

If the stomach reflex is out of balance, consider:

Physical prompts:

- Are they aware of any issues with their stomach?

- Have they had any nausea or vomiting recently?

- Do they ever get a sour, unpleasant taste in their mouth?

- Do they get 'butterflies' in their tummy when they are stressed?

- Have they changed their diet recently?

N.B. Also consider if there is anything in their lifestyle which may be causing inflammation or irritation in the stomach lining (but as yet is asymptomatic) such as excessive alcohol consumption, regular use of Aspirin, Ibuprofen or other non-steroidal anti-inflammatory drugs (NSAIDs). This will have to be handled sensitively (especially if there is excessive alcohol consumption); judge how well you know your client and then consider a phrase such as:

- *It may be that the painkillers you are on are causing a little irritation – do you always take these after you have eaten?*

- *You mentioned your alcohol consumption is quite high and alcohol can irritate the stomach lining, which is possibly what I am picking up.*

Liver

Location in the body

The liver is located in the upper right section of the abdomen, below the diaphragm. The liver is the second largest organ after the skin and weighs nearly 1.5kg. It is approximately triangular in shape and extends across the right hand side of the body.

Location on the feet

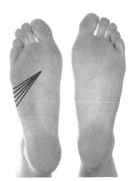

The liver is found on the right foot below the diaphragm line and is worked as a triangle with the point just resting over the stomach reflex.

Location on the hands

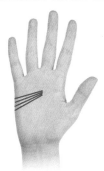

Right hand only - Thumb walk or knuckle down below the diaphragm line in Zones 5 - 2, three quarters of the way down palm.

Physiological action of the liver

The liver has an estimated 500 different functions, but in terms of digestion it is responsible for producing bile, which is then passed into the gall bladder. The liver is made of soft tissue surrounded by a connective tissue capsule. This capsule is further covered and reinforced by the peritoneum of the abdominal cavity, which protects the liver and holds it in place within the abdomen.

The blood supply of the liver is unique due to the hepatic portal vein system. As blood passes through the spleen, stomach, pancreas, gall bladder and intestines, it collects in the hepatic portal vein and is only then returned to the heart via the vena cava.

The liver consists of 4 distinct lobes - the left, right, caudate, and quadrate lobes - and about 60% of the liver is made up of hepatocytes (cells which absorb nutrients and remove harmful substances from the blood). It is estimated that the liver has over 500 functions, with the main functions including:

- processing digested food from the intestine.
- controlling levels of fats, amino acids and glucose in the blood.
- combating infections in the body through the macrophage system.
- clearing the blood of particles and infections including bacteria that cannot be removed via the kidneys.
- neutralising and destroying drugs and toxins.
- manufacturing bile.
- storing iron, vitamins and other essential chemicals.
- breaking down food and production of energy.
- storage and release of glycogen when energy is required quickly.
- manufacturing, breaking down and regulating numerous hormones including sex hormones.
- making enzymes and proteins which are responsible for most chemical reactions in the body, for example those involved in blood clotting and repair of damaged tissues.

In terms of the digestion, the liver has an active role by producing bile (a mixture of water, bile salts, cholesterol and bilirubin), which is produced by the hepatocytes. Bile then passes through the bile ducts to be stored in the gall bladder. When food containing fats reaches the duodenum, the cells of the duodenum release the hormone cholecystokinin to stimulate the gall bladder to release bile. Bile is released into the duodenum where it emulsifies large accumulations of fat. Emulsification breaks down fats into smaller pieces which are easier for the body to digest.

Physical problems or illnesses to be aware of:

When thinking of the liver, it is important to think of all the issues that might affect it and check to see if there are any present now, or whether there have been any problems in the past.

Cirrhosis - Irreversible scarring of the liver. Healthy liver tissue is destroyed and replaced by scar tissue, which starts to block the flow of blood through the liver, thus reducing liver function. This is usually caused by excessive alcohol consumption or the hepatitis C virus. Less common causes include hepatitis B, inherited liver disease, non-alcoholic steatohepatitis and autoimmune hepatitis.

Hepatitis - Inflammation of the liver, usually caused by a virus. Sometimes in mild cases it is asymptomatic and the person may not even be aware that they are infected, successfully fighting off the virus. In others, hepatitis can cause irreversible liver damage. If the hepatitis is acute or severe then common symptoms can include: right sided abdominal pain, nausea, fever, weight loss, tiredness and jaundice.

Jaundice - Yellow discoloration of the skin and the whites of the eyes. It is a symptom of disease, not a condition itself. The body fluids may also appear discoloured. Depending on the cause of the jaundice, symptoms may also include tiredness, abdominal pain, itchy skin, vomiting, weight loss and fever.

Jaundice results from excessively high levels of a yellowish pigment called bilirubin in the blood. Bilirubin originates in the red blood cells. The liver breaks down bilirubin and excretes it. If for any reason the liver cannot remove the bilirubin, jaundice occurs.

Remember to state that reflexology is a sensitive therapy that can pick up current issues and past issues – it does not mean there are any major problems and may relate to a physical or an emotional imbalance in the body.

If the liver reflex is out of balance, consider:

Physical prompts:

- Are they aware of any issues with their liver?

- Has there been a change in the amount of alcohol they have drunk recently?

- Have they had any infections recently, especially of the digestive system?

- Have they made any changes to their diet, especially of fatty foods?

- Have they increased their physical activity? *This may mean the liver is having to release more energy.*

- Are they on medications which may be broken down by the liver?

Gall bladder

Location in the body

The gall bladder is a small hollow organ that lies just below the right lobe of the liver and measures approximately 8x4cm when distended. The gall bladder narrows at the end closest to the liver into a small bile duct known as the cystic duct. The cystic duct connects to the common hepatic duct that carries bile from the liver. These ducts merge to form the common bile duct that extends to the wall of the duodenum.

Location on the feet

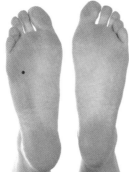

Right foot only - The gall bladder is commonly placed at the base of the 4th metatarsal, just below the diaphragm line. If the toes are flexed back the base of the metatarsal can be easily felt. Push up and turn onto the base of the bone.

Location on the hands

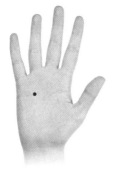

Right hand only - Push in and rotate at the base of the 4th metacarpal, just below the diaphragm line.

Physiological action of the gall bladder

The gall bladder stores bile received from the liver until it is needed for the digestion of fatty foods in the duodenum. Bile is produced by hepatocyte cells in the liver and passes through the bile ducts to the cystic duct. Bile is then pushed into the gall bladder by peristalsis. Water is absorbed through the walls of the gall bladder to concentrate the bile. The gall bladder stores this concentrated bile until it is needed for digestion.

When chyme passes through the pyloric sphincter into the duodenum, if fats or proteins are detected, sensory receptors in the walls of the duodenum respond by producing the hormone cholecystokinin (CKK). The CKK enters the blood stream and travels to the gall bladder. Here it stimulates the smooth muscle tissue of the gall bladder to contract. This forces the bile out into the cystic duct, into the common bile duct and out into the duodenum, where it breaks up the fats for easier digestion by the pancreatic juices.

Physical problems or illnesses to be aware of:

When thinking of the gall bladder, it is important to think of all the issues that might affect it and check to see if there are any present now, or whether there have been any problems in the past.

Gallstones - Small stones that form in the gall bladder. It is thought that gallstones develop due to an imbalance in the chemical composition of bile. Gallstones are commonly made up of cholesterol and so a diet high in cholesterol may be a cause. Risk factors include age (more common around the age of 40), sex (women are more likely to develop stones), obesity, cirrhosis and family history.

Remember to state that reflexology is a sensitive therapy that can pick up current issues and past issues – it does not mean there are any major problems and may relate to a physical or an emotional imbalance in the body.

If the gall bladder reflex is out of balance, consider:

Physical prompts:

- Are they aware of any issues with their gall bladder?

- Has there been a change in their diet, especially an increase in fatty foods?

- Do they feel uncomfortable after eating fatty foods?

Pancreas

Location in the body

The pancreas is a long narrow organ (6 -10cm long) that lies behind the stomach on the left side of the abdominal cavity. The head of the pancreas connects to the duodenum and the tail of the pancreas extends to the left side of the abdominal cavity, near the spleen.

The pancreas also has an endocrine function (see page 48) as well as producing digestive enzymes.

Location on the feet

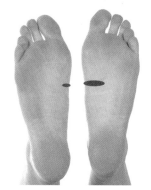

Thumb walk under the ball of the foot in Zone 1 on the right foot and Zones 1 and 2 of the left.

Location on the hands

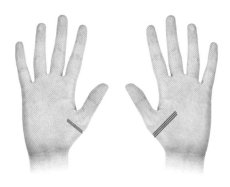

Thumb walk just below the base of the thumb on the right hand and at the base of thumb and first finger on the left.

Physiological action of the pancreas

The stomach slowly releases partially digested food (chyme) into the duodenum, where enzymes produced by the pancreas (called pancreatic juice) complete digestion. Pancreatic juice is a mixture of water, salts, bicarbonate and many different digestive enzymes. The bicarbonate ions neutralize the acid in chyme, allowing the enzymes to function correctly and protecting the walls of the duodenum. The enzymes found in pancreatic juice have different digestive functions:

- Pancreatic amylase breaks large polysaccharides like starches and glycogen into smaller sugars such as maltose, maltotriose, and glucose.

- Trypsin, chymotrypsin, and carboxypeptidase break proteins down into their amino acid subunits.

- Pancreatic lipase breaks large triglyceride molecules into fatty acids and monoglycerides.

- Ribonuclease and deoxyribonuclease digest nucleic acids. Ribonuclease breaks down molecules of RNA, whilst Deoxyribonuclease digests DNA molecules.

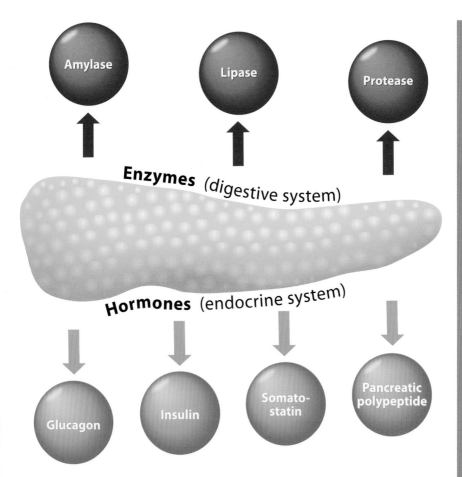

Physical problems or illnesses to be aware of:

When thinking of the pancreas, it is important to think of all the issues that might affect it and check to see if there are any present now, or whether there have been any problems in the past.

Pancreatitis - a serious condition where the pancreas becomes inflamed; this can be acute or chronic. Signs and symptoms of pancreatitis include severe pain in the upper abdomen and back, nausea and vomiting. If it is acute pancreatitis, there is often a fever; with chronic pancreatitis, there may be weight loss and diarrhoea.

The most common causes of acute pancreatitis are gallstones, heavy alcohol use or trauma. Chronic pancreatitis may develop as a result of acute pancreatitis but it is most commonly due to many years of alcohol abuse.

Pancreatic cancer - the fourth most common cause of cancer death in men and the fifth in women. One of the major challenges associated with pancreatic cancer is that signs and symptoms seldom occur until advanced stages. By the time symptoms occur, cancer cells are likely to have spread (metastasised) to other parts of the body, often preventing surgical removal of tumours.

Remember to state that reflexology is a sensitive therapy that can pick up current issues and past issues – it does not mean there are any major problems and may relate to a physical or an emotional imbalance in the body.

If the pancreas reflex is out of balance, this could be due to either endocrine (see page 48) or exocrine issues, consider:

Physical prompts:

- Do they get any right sided abdominal pain?
- Do they get regular nausea, vomiting or had any weight loss?
- Are they aware if they have any problems with blood sugar levels?
- Has their diet changed, especially changes to the amount of sugar they eat?
- Do they ever feel like they could faint when they haven't eaten?
- Do they go to the loo more than usual?
- Do they have any problems with their digestive system?

N.B. these could be symptoms of a medical problem, so advise your client to take these symptoms to their GP where they might be offered further tests.

Small intestine

Location in body

The small intestine follows on from the stomach. It is a long, twisting, hollow tube approximately 4 - 6m long. It is only about 2.5cm in diameter, which is why it is known as the small intestine. It is found throughout the abdominal cavity and lies anterior to the stomach, continuing down into the top of the pelvic cavity. It is divided into three separate parts:

- The duodenum is the smallest section (approximately 30cm) of the small intestine; it is C-shaped and lies adjacent to the stomach.

- The jejunum is the middle section of the small intestine and is approximately 2.5m long, winding through the abdominal cavity.

- The last section is called the ileum which is 2 - 4m long. This sits in the lower abdominal cavity and ends at the ileo-caecal valve.

Location on the feet

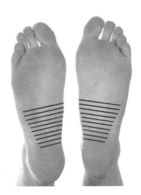

Located from under the diaphragm line down to the redness of the heel.

Location on the hands

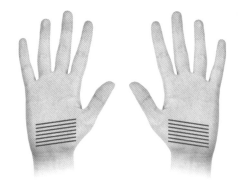

This area is the lower third of the palm of each hand. Use 2 or 3 of your knuckles to claw across this area or thumb walk.

Physiological action of the small intestine

As the acidic chyme enters the duodenum from the stomach (through the pyloric sphincter), the Brunner's glands secrete mucous which contains bicarbonate, an alkaline, to neutralize the chyme. This prevents the stomach acid from damaging the duodenum and provides a neutral pH to optimize the work of enzymes in the next stage of chemical digestion.

The chyme at this stage still contains partially digested food and as this enters the duodenum it causes the liver to produce bile and the gall bladder to release it into the duodenum. It also causes the pancreas to produce pancreatic juices. Bile acts as an emulsifier for fats, breaking up lipids to increase their surface area. The pancreatic juice contains enzymes which can break down carbohydrates, lipids and proteins into their smallest components ready for absorption. The peristaltic action of the duodenum ensures that all the chyme is mixed with the enzymes until the chemical digestion is completed on the chyme.

Peristalsis (the involuntary constriction and relaxation of the muscles of the intestine, creating wave-like movements which push the contents forward) then slowly moves the digested chyme on to the jejunum, which is responsible for the majority of absorption of nutrients such as fructose, amino acids, small peptides, vitamins and most glucose.

The chyme then moves through to the ileum where remaining nutrients are absorbed before the chyme passes on to the large intestine. Amino acids and glucose produced by digestion are passed into the hepatic portal vein, and fatty acids and glycerol are passed into the lacteals (small lymph vessels). The ileum also has Peyer's patches, which are lymphoid tissue to protect against any bacteria or viruses in the chyme.

Physical problems or illnesses to be aware of:

When thinking of the small intestine, it is important to think of all the issues that might affect it and check to see if there are any present now, or whether there have been any problems in the past.

Coeliac disease - a common digestive condition where a person has an adverse reaction to gluten. It is an autoimmune condition.

Crohn's disease - a chronic inflammatory disease that can affect any part of the digestive tract, but most commonly the ileum. It may be caused by a malfunction in the immune system, causing the body to attack "friendly bacteria" in the intestines.

Duodenal ulcers – see peptic ulcers (stomach).

Irritable Bowel Syndrome - not a disease as such - it is diagnosed when there is no visible disease or damage to the intestinal wall but the patient has recurring symptoms of abdominal pain, cramping, and excess gas with either constipation or diarrhoea.

Remember to state that reflexology is a sensitive therapy that can pick up current issues and past issues – it does not mean there are any major problems and may relate to a physical or an emotional imbalance in the body.

If the small intestine reflex is out of balance, consider:

Physical prompts:

- Have they had any problems with their bowels recently?

- Are they prone to constipation or diarrhoea?

- Have they changed their diet recently?

- When they are stressed does it affect their bowels?

- Do they ever feel bloated?

- Do they sit for long periods with a poor posture, which may be affecting the nerve supply to the intestines?

N.B. Also consider if there is anything in their lifestyle which may be causing inflammation or irritation in the small intestine but as yet is asymptomatic, such as poor diet (lack of fibre, fatty or fried foods, processed foods etc).

This may be a time to address their diet, especially if they are feeling tired or stressed.

Appendix

Location in body

The appendix is a pouch-like structure that is connected to the caecum at the junction between the small and large intestines, below the ileo-caecal valve. It is located in the lower abdomen (iliac region) on the right hand side. It is approximately 10cm long and less than 1cm in diameter.

Location on the feet

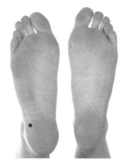

Located on the right foot on the redness of the heel in between Zones 4 and 5.

Location on the hands

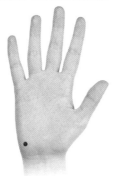

Located on the right hand just above the wrist in between Zones 4 and 5.

Physiological action of the appendix

The exact function of the appendix is unknown. It is thought that the appendix is probably an organ that now has no particular function as a result of our evolution. It certainly is not a vital organ and can be removed surgically if need be.

However it does contain lymphoid tissue so it is thought it may possibly have a minor role in the immune system. It may also store intestinal bacteria, so if needed it can re-colonise the intestines with good bacteria to help restore a healthy gut (e.g. after an episode of diarrhoea).

Physical problems or illnesses to be aware of:

When thinking of the appendix, it is important to think of all the issues that might affect it and check to see if there are any present now, or whether there have been any problems in the past.

Appendicitis - Inflammation of the appendix. The appendix becomes filled with bacteria that produce pus, causing the appendix to swell. This can be caused by infection (e.g. a stomach infection) or an obstruction (e.g. hard piece of faeces) in the appendix that causes a bacterial infection. Sometimes the cause is unknown.

Grumbling appendix - Whilst acute appendicitis needs medical attention and the client would have severe right lower abdominal pain, there is some debate as to whether there is such a thing as chronic appendicitis or 'grumbling appendix'. Whilst the jury is out on this, there are many anecdotal tales of people who have complained of discomfort on the right side of their abdomen for many years, eventually develop acute appendicitis, and then the previous discomfort never returns.

Remember to state that reflexology is a sensitive therapy that can pick up current issues and past issues – it does not mean there are any major problems and may relate to a physical or an emotional imbalance in the body.

If the appendix reflex is out of balance, consider:

Physical prompts:

- Do they get any dull aches or sharp pains on the right side of their abdomen?

- Do they sit for long periods with a poor posture, which may be affecting the nerve supply to the abdominal area?

N.B. It is essential to reassure clients that an imbalance here does not mean that they have appendicitis, but may just indicate a minor irritation in or around the appendix or ileocaecal valve.

If the pain remains constant or becomes more acute they should be referred to a GP. Tell your client to make an appointment with their GP to discuss their symptoms. Reassure them that this is probably something minor but is worth checking out.

Large intestine

Location in body

The large intestine is the last part of the intestinal tract and is located around the borders of the abdominal cavity. It starts on the lower right hand side near the iliac crest, and then moves up towards the liver (ascending colon) where it turns at a right angle (hepatic flexure) to cross the body (transverse colon). When it reaches the spleen, it turns at a right angle again (splenic flexure) to travel down the left hand side of the abdominal cavity (descending colon). At the end of the descending colon, the large intestine turns slightly medially at the sigmoid flexure to form the S-shaped sigmoid colon before entering into the rectum.

The large intestine is approximately 1.5m in length and although it is shorter than the small intestine, it is a wider tube, at approximately 7cm in diameter.

Location on the feet

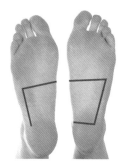

On the right foot, walk up from the redness of the heel. Then cross the foot, remaining under the liver and stomach reflexes. Continue across the left foot and turn to walk down to the redness of the heel. Then turn again to walk along the redness of the heel.

Location on the hands

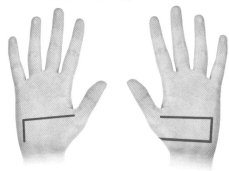

The large intestine can be found in the lower third of both hands. The easiest way to work this is to use your knuckles to work in a circular motion in a clockwise direction, as this mimics the way the large intestine flows.

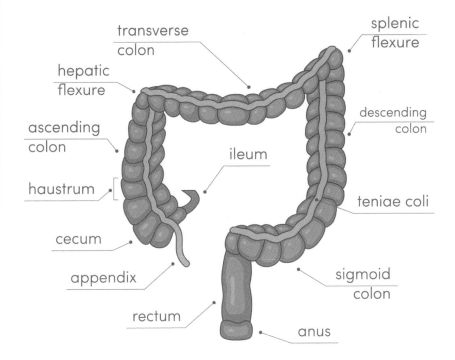

transverse colon

splenic flexure

hepatic flexure

ascending colon

descending colon

ileum

haustrum

teniae coli

cecum

appendix

sigmoid colon

rectum

anus

Physiological action of the colon

The main function of the large intestine is to absorb water and vitamins. By removing water, the chyme becomes more solid to form faeces. Watery chyme enters the caecum through the ileo-caecal valve, where it is mixed with intestinal bacteria. Peristalsis then continues to move the chyme through the whole of the large intestine; this can take several hours. The bacteria begin to digest substances that cannot be digested higher up in the gastrointestinal (GI) tract and as a result are able to release many vitamins including vitamins K, B1, B2, B6 and B12. Gases such as carbon dioxide and methane are also produced as a by-product of bacterial fermentation and may lead to flatulence.

Water is also absorbed in the large intestine to help maintain fluid levels in the body and as a result, more solid faeces is produced. This is then stored in the rectum and sigmoid colon before elimination.

Physical problems or illnesses to be aware of:

When thinking of the large intestine, it is important to think of all the issues that might affect it and check to see if there are any present now, or whether there have been any problems in the past.

Crohn's disease - A chronic inflammatory disease that can affect any part of the digestive tract (see small intestine on page 85).

Diarrhoea - The passing of frequent, loose watery stools. Diarrhoea may be accompanied by abdominal pain, bloating, loss of appetite and vomiting. Can lead to dehydration, causing headache, weakness and lethargy.

Diverticulitis - The inflammation of small pouches known as diverticula in the wall of the colon causes the symptoms associated with this disease. Often associated with persistent constipation and pain.

Flatulence - Passing of gas from the digestive system out of the anus.

Gastroenteritis - Inflammation of the lining of the stomach and intestines.

Ulcerative Colitis - Chronic intermittent inflammation and ulceration of the colon. The lining of the colon becomes inflamed, swollen and ulcerates. The ulcers can bleed and create mucous and pus.

Remember to state that reflexology is a sensitive therapy that can pick up current issues and past issues – it does not mean there are any major problems and may relate to a physical or an emotional imbalance in the body.

If the large intestine reflex is out of balance, consider:

Physical prompts:

- Have they had any problems with their bowels recently?

- Are they prone to constipation or diarrhoea?

- Have they changed their diet recently? *Even if they have improved their diet it can take time for the digestive system to become used to this.*

- When they are stressed does it tend to affect their bowels?

- Do they ever feel bloated?

- Do they sit for long periods, with a poor posture, which may be affecting the nerve supply to the intestines?

Rectum/anus

Location in body

The rectum is a short, muscular tube that forms the lowest portion of the large intestine and connects the sigmoid colon to the anus. It is approximately 12cm long, lying inferior to the sacral spine and connecting to the anus, the passage through the pelvic floor.

Location on the feet

There are two common placements:

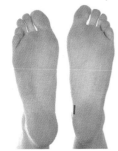

1. The first placement is on the left foot, on the plantar aspect in Zone 1, working from the redness of the heel down.

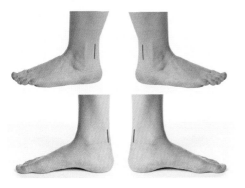

2. The second placement is at the back of the heel. The thumb and finger squeeze either side of the Achilles tendon behind the ankle bone.

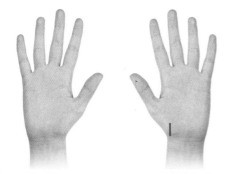

Location on the hands

Left hand only - at the base of the thumb in Zone 1, work down to the wrist line.

Physiological action of the rectum/anus

Faeces collect in the rectum and in the lower sigmoid colon, which act as temporary storage areas until there is enough pressure on the rectal walls to cause nerve impulses to pass messages to the brain. This then contracts the voluntary muscles in the anus, alerting the individual of the need to defecate. The rectum then shortens and forces the faeces into the anal canal. Peristalsis propels it out of the rectum, opening the internal and external sphincter muscles of the anus and allowing the faeces to exit the body.

Physical problems or illnesses to be aware of:

When thinking of the rectum and anus, it is important to think of all the issues that might affect them and check to see if there are any present now, or whether there have been any problems in the past.

Constipation - The infrequent, difficult or incomplete emptying of the bowel which leads to hard faeces. Can be caused by a number (and often a combination) of factors including insufficient fibre and fluids in the diet, changes in routine and eating habits, lack of exercise and immobility, ignoring the urge to defecate, and anxiety and depression.

Haemorrhoids - Swollen veins inside the rectum and around the anus, commonly called piles. There are two main types; internal (occurring inside the rectum) and external (occurring outside the rectum). Internal haemorrhoids are more common.

Rectal prolapse - the protrusion of the rectum into the anus or external area. Commonly caused by a weakened pelvic floor after childbirth.

Remember to state that reflexology is a sensitive therapy that can pick up current issues and past issues – it does not mean there are any major problems and may relate to a physical or an emotional imbalance in the body.

If the rectum/anus reflex is out of balance, consider:

Physical prompts:

- Are they prone to constipation?

- Do they have any pain when they open their bowels?

- Do they have, or have they ever suffered with piles/haemorrhoids?

- (If a the client is a woman with children) Did they have any issues with piles during pregnancy?

Emotional links: digestive system

If these physical issues are present, the emotional involvement may still be important as part of the illness. If none of these are present then it is even more important to consider emotional blocks.

Key areas: how you digest life; from the mouth to the anus, the absorption of life takes place. How it is processed, which elements are retained and which are let go of is represented in the digestive system.

The function of the whole digestive system from the mouth to the anus is to take in nourishment from the food that we eat and process it. This can be likened to life – it represents how you take in life and process life, life issues, life joys, etc. It is related to how the person filters and processes life and what life presents us. If there are digestive issues, they represent the emotional problems and areas that are there for improving, resolving or learning about. Often reflexology imbalances are about awareness and family programming. Each family has its own way of living and children learn a great deal about life according to what their parents teach them, show by example and what they say. This becomes family programming. Many people say that digestive issues are common in their family; however, it may be that the ways of thinking and learned behaviours on how to live, what to say or not to say, how to act/ not to act etc, are actually the potentially corrupt programmes that lead to the digestive issues.

95

Physically, this system is where the body takes what it needs and moves everything else on. In life, this can be a healthy system or not. Some people know what is good for them and some do not, e.g. saying 'yes' when they mean 'no' and doing things that they would rather not do.

Be aware as you listen, not to tell them how you think they should move forward, but instead ask useful questions to allow them to explore the ideas.

Exploring possible emotional reasons for reflexes that are out of balance has to be handled with great sensitivity, and it can be presented purely as one school of thought. It may be that it is not suitable to share this information with your client, but it might help you understand why the reflex is imbalanced. You will need to use careful judgement as to whether to share this information.

The mouth: *what we take in and reject in communication terms.*

- Are they speaking up, putting their view forward?
- Are they swallowing any situation because they believe they can't change it?
- Is there something they could do to change it?
- Are they able to express easily their core beliefs and ideas?
- Are they speaking their truths and values or someone else's?

The stomach: *how we stomach or cope with life and start to absorb and "chew life over" – a process started with chewing in the mouth.*

- Is there something that they are finding difficult to stomach?
- Was there a situation in their past that was difficult to stomach?

The liver: *this is about keeping in anger about something.*

- Have there have been any situations recently where they have felt angry?
- Have they ever felt that they had to suppress their anger?

The gall bladder: *this is about making decisions.*

- Are they having trouble making a decision about something?
- Do they have too many decisions to make?

The pancreas: *all about the sweetness of life (or not). Digesting life and creating the sweet balance of life.*

- Have they felt the sweetness disappearing from their life recently?
- Was there a situation in the past when they felt that sweetness was drained from their life?

The general intestinal area

- How are things at home for the client?

- Are there issues to do with their family or private life?

- Are they walking the easiest path that perhaps doesn't exactly fit them?

The small intestine: *all about the absorption of life; this also sits in the area of family and home, so there may be cross references to home issues.*

- Are they finding something difficult to absorb?

- Are they hanging on to something that they should let go of?

The ascending colon: *this area is about taking up life, of beginning to process life, to be able to process and filter /digest and then be creatively themselves.*

- Is there anything they are having problems with in their life?

- Are they feeling stagnated creatively?

- Can they be the person they feel they really are?

- Have they had problems in the past in moving forward and taking the next steps?

The transverse colon: *this area is about honouring the self, of being creative, of being courageous and able to cope with life shocks (or not!)*

- Do they need to be brave about something to feel really themselves?

The descending colon: *this area is about staying grounded; being able to physically process and let go of what is not helpful to each unique individual and the person that only they can be in the world.*

- Do they have emotions that need to be released or let go? *If so, then to let go will be healing. Note: they may need to visit a counsellor/ their GP for help in doing this.*

The rectum/anus: *to do with sense of security and plans for the future.*

- Are they feeling insecure about their plans for the future?

The Musculo-skeletal System

Introduction

The musculo-skeletal system comprises two groups of bodily structures: muscles and bones. Without this system, the human body would not hold the shape it does, but instead be a soft, shapeless mass of flesh on the floor.

This system gives the human body shape, form and support, allowing us to look the way we do and to hold ourselves in an upright position. It protects the softer, more easily damaged organs beneath it and allows the body to move independently. Bones also store minerals such as calcium, and have a role connected to the circulatory system, as the bone marrow is where blood cells are produced.

This is one of the larger and more structurally complex systems of the body, comprising 206 bones in an adult body and between 640 and 840 named muscles, depending on which source you read. However, to make things more manageable, these have been grouped into the sections of the body that can easily be found as reflexology points.

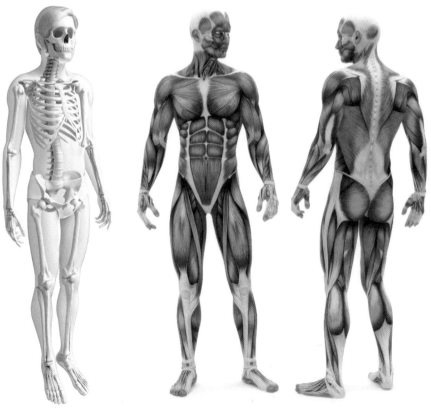

The head

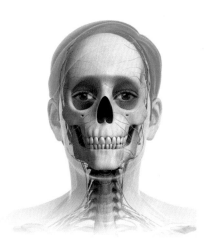

Location in body

The head is located at the top (the most superior part) of the body. The head is often regarded in two sections; the face and the cranial part of the skull.

Location on the feet:

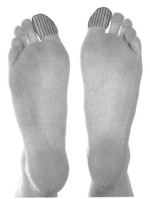

On the plantar aspect of the feet, thumb walk vertically over the most distal section of the big toe on both aspects, being careful over the nail. Finish with a thumb walk covering the sides and tip of the toe to the first joint.

Location on the hands:

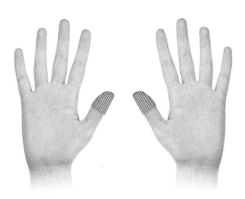

Thumb walk over the most lateral section of the client's thumb on both anterior and posterior sides, being careful of their nail. Finish with a thumb walk around from one side at the knuckle joint, up to the tip and round to the other side at the knuckle joint.

Physiological action

The skull is made up of 8 cranial bones and 14 facial bones. These are held together by cartilage. The skull protects the brain and sensory organs, as well as facilitating eating (via the jaw and teeth). The bones of the skull also provide attachment sites for the muscles of the face and head.

The muscles of the head allow for facial expression and movement of the head; they also keep the head upright, facilitate the chewing action and help our hair stand on end!

Physical problems or illnesses to be aware of:

When thinking of the head, it is important to think of all the issues that might affect it and check to see if there are any present now, or whether there have been any problems with this area in the past.

Some examples might be:

Bell's palsy – this is temporary partial or complete weakness or paralysis of the muscles of the face. It normally affects just one side of the face, although in some rare cases it can affect both sides. It is caused by the facial nerve becoming compressed or inflamed.

Fractures - when the bone breaks, usually from impact.

Headaches - these can come in a number of different varieties, and we shall only look at primary headaches (not caused by any other condition) here. The most common form is tension headaches, which can feel like a dull ache with constant pressure around the front, top and sides of the head. Another less common form is cluster headaches, which is intense pain which is usually located behind one eye, which will happen frequently for a time and then stop for a time (they happen in cycles).

Migraines - sudden, debilitating headaches, which may be preceded by visual disturbances, anxiety, mood swings, changes in energy levels, co-ordination problems, speech difficulties, muscular stiffness or tingling in the neck and shoulders and an altered sense of taste and smell.

Tetanus – one of the most common symptoms of tetanus is lockjaw, which is stiffness and spasming in the muscles of the jaw. This is caused by the neurotoxin produced by bacteria that would most likely have entered into the body elsewhere, usually through a cut or severe burn.

Tooth disorders – from toothache to tooth decay, to abscesses beneath the teeth, tooth disorders can not only bring pain to the area of the teeth, but also to the cheekbone area and even up into the head causing headaches.

Temporomandibular joint (TMJ) disorders - issues that affect the joint between the skull and the lower jaw. Symptoms may include clicking, popping or grating noises as the client chews, muscle spasms in the jaw area, pain that starts in front of the ear but may spread out to the temple, the cheek or the ear, earache, headache or a tight jaw or difficulty with opening the mouth.

Remember that some of the muscles that attach to the skull can have an effect much lower down the body due to their other connections and attachments. For example, the trapezius muscle attaches at the base of the skull – but its other attachments are in each shoulder and the mid-back. Problems and tightness in this muscle could cause neck ache, tightness across the shoulders, back ache or even headache due to the muscles being drawn tight across the skull. There are other muscles like this, so it is worth looking in more depth when faced with a problem in the upper body to see if its connections can reach as high as the head and thus cause seemingly unrelated symptoms like headaches.

Other common problems that may affect the area:

Acne - a chronic skin disease that affects nearly all adolescents to some extent, causing small spots or lumps to be present on the skin (most commonly on the face, back or chest).

Alopecia - sudden, often temporary, hair loss.

Dandruff - a common condition that affects the skin of the scalp, which causes small (but visible) flakes of skin to shed.

Folliculitis - most commonly caused by bacteria infecting pre-existing damage to the hair follicle (e.g. friction, shaving, insect bites or a blocked follicle) and is characterised by itchy or painful redness, with small red pimples in the upper part of the follicles which may crust over. This is called Barber's Itch when found on the beard area of the face. Folliculitis can be found in any hairy area of the body, not just the face or scalp.

A mouth ulcer - an open sore on the lining of the mouth.

Remember to state that reflexology is a sensitive therapy that can pick up current issues and past issues – it does not mean there are any major problems and may relate to a physical or an emotional imbalance in the body.

If the head reflex is out of balance, consider:

Physical prompts:

- Have they had a headache recently or is this something that they tend to suffer with?

- Do they carry tension in their neck, as this can also cause tension in the head area?

- Have they been under a lot of stress recently?

- Do they have a busy brain?

- Have they had a cold recently? *(especially if sinus reflexes come up)*

- Have they been on a long haul flight? *Aircraft pressure can change how these function (especially if the sinus/ eustacian tube reflexes come up).*

- Have they had any dizziness recently or issues with their ears? *(especially if the eustacian tubes and ear reflexes are out of balance).*

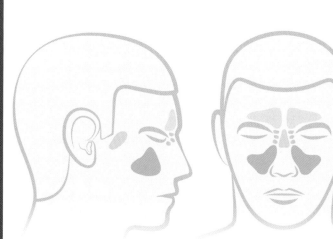

Paranasal sinuses

Frontal sinuses

Ethmoidal sinuses

Sphenoidal sinuses

Maxillary sinuses

The neck

Location in body

The neck joins the head to the trunk of the body, allowing for movement of the head and providing a pathway for the spinal cord, the oesophagus and the trachea.

Location on the feet:

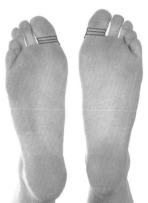

Work both the plantar and dorsal aspects of the feet. Walk across the base of the big toes. Distal to the metatarsophalangeal joint.

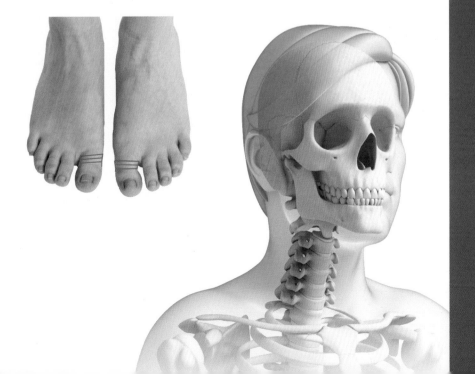

Location on the hands:

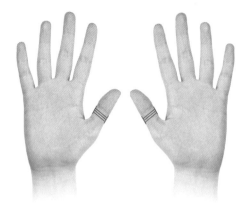

Work both the palmar and dorsal aspects of the hands. Walk across the thumb, proximal to the first joint.

Physiological action

The neck contains seven irregular-shaped bones that are part of the vertebral column, called the cervical vertebrae. These are sandwiched together by cartilage discs. Through the middle of the cervical vertebrae, there is a hole through which the spinal cord runs. The bones of the vertebrae protect the spinal cord, which is part of the central nervous system, as well as allowing rotation, flexion (both anterior and from side to side), and extension.

The muscles of the neck produce the movement of the neck and head, as well as keeping the head upright to provide a clear path for trachea and oesophagus.

Physical problems or illnesses to be aware of:

When thinking of the neck, it is important to think of all the issues that might affect it and check to see if there are any present now, or whether there have been problems with this area in the past.

Some examples might be:

Torticollis (also known as a 'wry neck') - a painful condition in which neck muscles contract involuntarily, causing the head to twist or turn to one side.

Whiplash - where the ligaments, tendons and muscles of the neck are damaged by a sudden movement of the head forwards, backwards or sideways.

Other common conditions that may affect this area are:

Laryngitis - inflammation of the larynx. This leads the larynx to be red and swollen, accompanied by a hoarseness or loss of voice, a sore throat, mild fever, a cough and a constant need to clear the throat.

Pharyngitis - commonly known as a sore throat.

Tonsillitis - an inflammation of the tonsils caused by either a bacterial or viral infection.

Some of the muscles that form the neck can have an effect much lower down the body due to their other connections and attachments, so it is worth looking at the reflexes for shoulder, back, head, hips and knees to see if the cause of the imbalance could originate somewhere else.

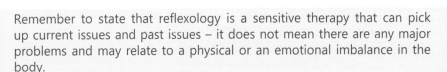

Remember to state that reflexology is a sensitive therapy that can pick up current issues and past issues – it does not mean there are any major problems and may relate to a physical or an emotional imbalance in the body.

If the neck reflex is out of balance, consider:

Physical prompts:

- Do they have any stiffness or pain in their neck?

- If they are stressed, do they carry their tension in their neck and shoulders?

- Do they sit at a computer for long periods – is their working position correct? *If they hunch over or look down at a keyboard, this can put strain on the neck muscles.*

- An imbalance in the neck reflex is common in times of high stress – might this be the reason?

- How would they describe their posture when they are sitting, standing and walking – is their head held upright with their shoulders back?

- Do they do any activities that involve them moving their neck repeatedly such as swimming? *Whilst swimming is very good exercise, if they swim with their head held out of the water. this places strain on the neck.*

- How do they answer their phone? *People often tilt their head to one side when answering a phone, which puts stress on the neck muscles when done regularly.*

- Do they carry a heavy bag on one shoulder?

The spine

Location on the feet:

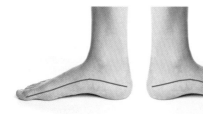

The spine is along the medial edge of the foot. Work down the inside of the foot on the bone.

Location on the hands:

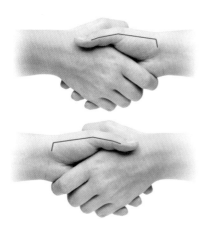

Shake hands with your client, rotate the hand so you can walk from the tip of the thumb to the base of the hand along the bone.

Physiological action:

The spine (or vertebral column) consists of 33 interlocking irregular bones called vertebrae, which are separated from each other by a cushion of cartilage. Each vertebra has a hole running through it through which the spinal cord (see page 157) passes.

The spine is split into five sections: seven cervical vertebrae (the neck), twelve thoracic vertebrae (the upper body), five lumbar vertebrae (the lower curve of the spine), five vertebrae fused together to form the sacrum (between the curve of the back and the tailbone), and four vertebrae fused together to form the coccyx (also known as the tailbone, which is at the lowest part of the spine).

The function of the spine is to protect the spinal cord, to support the structure and weight of the body in certain activities, to provide attachment points for the ribs, pelvic bones and some skeletal muscles, and to provide balance, stability, flexibility and mobility through the length of the upper body. Its S-shaped overall structure gives maximum shock absorption during everyday activities such as walking, running, jumping etc.

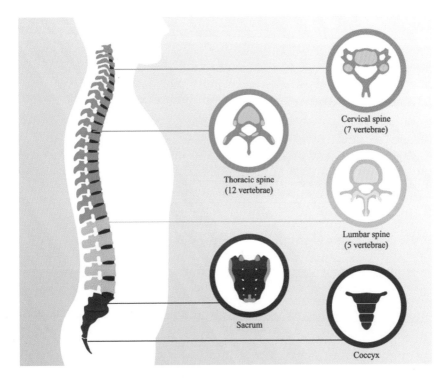

Cervical spine
(7 vertebrae)

Thoracic spine
(12 vertebrae)

Lumbar spine
(5 vertebrae)

Sacrum

Coccyx

Physical problems or illnesses to be aware of:

When thinking of the spine, it is important to think of all the issues that might affect it and check to see if there are any present now, or whether there have been any problems in this area in the past.

Arthritis - can take one of two forms. Rheumatoid arthritis is an autoimmune condition, where the body's immune system attacks the body. Common symptoms are hot, red, swollen joints and stiffness through the joint. Osteoarthritis is simply wear and tear on the joint that commonly causes pain, stiffness and knobbly or crackly joints.

Kyphosis - where the outward curvature at the top of the thoracic part of the spine is excessive, resulting in a rounded back or 'hunchback'.

Lordosis - where there is an excessive inward curvature of the lumbar spine.

Prolapsed intevertebral disc - where the gelatinous inner layer of the intevertebral disc (cartilage) protrudes out of the spinal column, distorting the shape of the disc. This can also lead the disc to rupture, or can put pressure on either an individual nerve or the spinal cord, which can lead to pain in whichever area of the body is served by that nerve.

Scoliosis - where there is an abnormal twisting and sideways curvature of the spine.

Paget's disease is, after osteoporosis, the second most common type of bone disease in the UK. It is where bone tissue is replaced at a faster rate than is normal, leading to enlarged, brittle bones. It most commonly affects the pelvis or the spine.

Remember to state that reflexology is a sensitive therapy that can pick up current issues and past issues – it does not mean there are any major problems and may relate to a physical or an emotional imbalance in the body.

If the spine reflex is out of balance, consider:

Physical prompts:

- Do they suffer from back ache/ neck problems/ shoulder ache?

- Have they had any back problems in the past?

- Do they tend to sit in one position for large parts of the day?

108

The shoulders

Location in body

The shoulders join the arms to the trunk of the body at the lateral superior corners of the main trunk of the body.

Location on the feet:

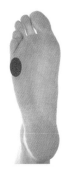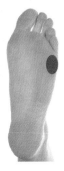

Work on the joint in zone 5 around the fifth metatarsal pharangeal joint just below the little toe.

Location on the hands:

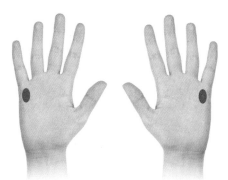

Work on the joint in zone 5, just below the little finger.

Physiological action of the muscles and bones of the shoulder

The shoulder joint contains three bones of different types held together by ligaments and muscles. Being a ball-and-socket joint, the bones and muscles of the shoulder combine to allow the full range of movement: flexion, extension, abduction, adduction, circumduction, medial rotation and lateral rotation of the arm.

Physical problems or illnesses to be aware of:

When thinking of the shoulders, it is important to think of all the issues that might affect them and check to see if there are any present now, or whether there have been any problems in this area in the past.

Some examples might be:

Arthritis - can take one of two forms. Rheumatoid arthritis is an autoimmune condition, where the body's immune system attacks the body. Common symptoms are hot, red, swollen joints and stiffness through the joint. Osteoarthritis is simply wear and tear on the joint that commonly causes pain, stiffness and knobbly or crackly joints.

Bursitis - the inflammation of the bursa (fluid filled sac under the skin usually found around joints), causing pain, inflammation and tenderness.

Shoulder dislocation - where the humerus has popped out of its socket and the supporting tissues are stretched and/or torn.

Fractured clavicle - where the collar bone breaks, usually after a fall onto the shoulder.

Frozen shoulder - also known as adhesive capsulitis or shoulder contracture. Usually, with this condition, there is shoulder pain for the first two to nine months, followed by increasing stiffness until movement of the upper arm is either very limited or ceases altogether.

Tendonitis - inflammation of a tendon or tendons causing pain that gets worse on moving the affected area, as well as a grating or crackling sensation, swelling, weakness in the affected area and a lump along the tendon.

Remember that some of the muscles of the shoulder can have an effect lower down the body due to their other connections and attachments, so it is worth looking in more depth when faced with a problem in the upper body as to whether its connections can reach as high as the head or as low as the mid-back and thus cause seemingly unrelated symptoms like pain in the shoulder.

Remember to state that reflexology is a sensitive therapy that can pick up current issues and past issues – it does not mean there are any major problems and may relate to a physical or an emotional imbalance in the body.

If the shoulder reflex is out of balance, consider:

Physical prompts:

- Do they or have they had any problems with their shoulders?

- Do they get any stiffness or pain in their shoulders?

- If they are stressed, do they carry their tension in their neck and shoulders?

- Do they sit at a computer for long periods – is their working position correct? *If they hunch over a keyboard, shoulders can become tense; it is important they regularly lift their head and pull their shoulders back.*

- Tense shoulders are common in times of high stress – could this be the reason for the imbalance?

- How would they describe their posture when they are sitting, standing and walking – is their head held upright with their shoulders back?

- Do they tend to carry a heavy bag on one shoulder?

The elbows

Location in body

The elbows are hinge joints; one is present on each arm. They join the upper arm to the lower arm.

Location on the feet:

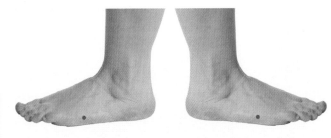

Push in and rotate halfway down the arm reflex on the lateral edge of the foot, in Zone 5.

Location on the hands:

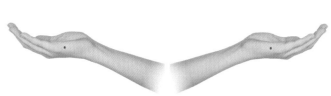

Push in and rotate halfway down the lateral edge of the hand, in Zone 5.

Physiological action

The elbow is the join between three bones; the humerus is in the upper arm, and the radius and ulna together make up the lower arm. As a hinge joint, it allows flexion and extension.

Physical problems or illnesses to be aware of:

When thinking of the elbows, it is important to think of all the issues that might affect them and check to see if there are any present now, or whether there have been any problems in this area in the past.

Classic examples would be:

Arthritis - can take one of two forms. Rheumatoid arthritis is an autoimmune condition, where the body's immune system attacks the body. Common symptoms are hot, red, swollen joints and stiffness through the joint. Osteoarthritis is simply wear and tear on the joint that commonly causes pain, stiffness and knobbly or crackly joints.

Bursitis is the inflammation of the bursa (fluid filled sac under the skin usually found around joints), causing pain, inflammation and tenderness.

Tennis elbow (if on the inside of the elbow) and *Golfers Elbow* (if on the outside of the elbow) are both the inflammation of a tendon at its attachment to one of the arm bones.

Remember to state that reflexology is a sensitive therapy that can pick up current issues and past issues – it does not mean there are any major problems and may relate to a physical or an emotional imbalance in the body.

If the elbow reflexes are out of balance, consider:

Physical prompts:

- Do they have or have they had any problems with their elbow?

- Do they or have they had any issues with their arm?

- Do they spend long periods of time on repetitive moves that involve bending the elbow, e.g. tennis or golf?

The sacro-iliac joint

Location in body

The Sacro-iliac joint (SIJ) is the joint between the pelvic bones (ilium) and the sacral bones of the spine.

Location on the feet:

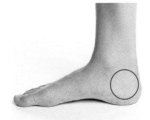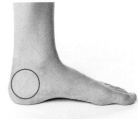

Located on the medial aspect of the foot, work over the calcaneus bone.

Location on the hands:

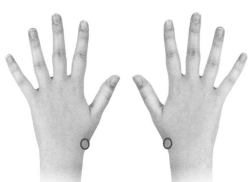

Located at the base of the thumb, work distal to the wrist.

Physiological action

The SIJ is a synovial plane joint where superficial ins and outs of the bones produce an interlocking joint which is reinforced by strong internal and external ligaments. These ligaments are so strong that the pelvic bones may fracture before the ligament breaks. Their main role is shock absorption, but also they help with the transfer of twisting motions in the lower body into the spine (torque conversion), and provide stability for the mechanical function of walking. There is the possibility in slippage in these joints from situations as small as stepping off a pavement incorrectly, resulting in the muscles around the pelvis tightening, which causes pain.

Physical problems or illnesses to be aware of:

When thinking of the sacroiliac joint, it is important to think of all the issues that might affect it and check to see if there are any present now, or whether there have been any problems in this area in the past.

114

Sacro-iliac joint dysfunction - dull lower back pain on both sides which might get worse on ascending stairs etc. In more severe situations there can be referred pain into the hip and groin and down the leg. This pain can be referred to the back and buttock and in rare situations down into the foot.

Sacroiliatis - inflammation of one or both SI joints resulting in pain in the back, buttocks or thighs.

Pregnancy - The SI joints relax under the action of the hormone Relaxin in pregnancy allowing the pelvic joints to widen for the birth process. This can lead to over-mobility which over years can result in osteoarthritis.

Remember to state that reflexology is a sensitive therapy that can pick up current issues and past issues – it does not mean there are any major problems and may relate to a physical or an emotional imbalance in the body.

If the sacroiliac joint reflex is out of balance, consider:

Physical prompts:

- Have they had any lower back or hip problems now or in the past?

- Have they had any slight slips or trips recently?

- Have they been pregnant?

The pelvis

Location in body

The pelvis meets the spine at the top of the sacral vertebrae, forms the hip bones, and circles around to the front (anterior) of the body to form the pubic bones, joined by the pubic symphysis (a small area of cartilage joining the pelvic bones). Together, it encircles the lower abdomen.

Location on the feet:

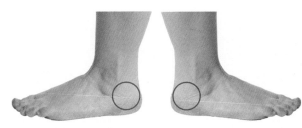

Massage around the back of the foot below the ankle.

Location on the hands:

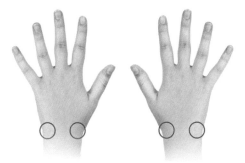

Massage around each wrist bone.

Physiological action

The pelvis performs two main functions: to protect the lower abdominal organs and to form ball-and-socket joints with both femur bones, allowing for free movement of the upper leg.

Physical problems or illnesses to be aware of:

When thinking of the pelvis, it is important to think of all the issues that might affect it and check to see if there are any present now, or whether there have been any problems in this area in the past.

Classic examples would be:

Arthritis - can take one of two forms. Rheumatoid arthritis is an autoimmune condition, where the body's immune system attacks the body. Common symptoms are hot, red, swollen joints and stiffness through the joint. Osteoarthritis is simply wear and tear on the joint that commonly causes pain, stiffness and knobbly or crackly joints.

Bursitis - the inflammation of the bursa (fluid filled sac under the skin usually found around joints), causing pain, inflammation and tenderness.

Dislocation - where the femur has popped out of its socket and the supporting tissues are stretched and/or torn.

Fractured hip - where the pelvic bone breaks, usually after a fall.

Osteoporosis - a condition that causes bones to become less dense and therefore weaker and more prone to fracture.

Paget's disease - after osteoporosis, this is the second most common type of bone disease in the UK. It is where bone tissue is replaced at a faster rate than is normal, leading to enlarged, brittle bones. It most commonly affects the pelvis or the spine.

Don't forget that some of the muscles of the hip and groin area can have an effect further up or lower down the body due to their other connections and attachments, so it is worth looking in more depth when faced with a problem in the lower body as to whether its connections could reach the hip or be caused by the changes in muscle use caused by a change in gait (the way one walks) or if the hip is weakened/hurting.

Remember to state that reflexology is a sensitive therapy that can pick up current issues and past issues – it does not mean there are any major problems and may relate to a physical or an emotional imbalance in the body.

If the pelvic reflex area is out of balance, consider:

Physical prompts:

- Do they have, or have they had, any problems with their pelvic area?

- Do they think this is an area where they hold tension? *A lot of people stand with their glutes tight and tense.*

- Do they have any problems with their digestion (bowels)?

- Do they have any problems with their periods? *Sometimes with heavy periods or issues with the uterus, the pelvic area may be tense.*

- Do they or have they had any issues with their lower back? *This may relate to tension in the pelvic girdle*

- Have they been doing exercise that might have affected their pelvis?

- If they had a pregnancy - did they have any back problems or pubic symphysis disorder?

The leg

Location in body

The leg is attached to the trunk of the body via the hip joint between the femur and the pelvis. It then runs vertically down, joining the foot at the ankle.

Location on the feet:

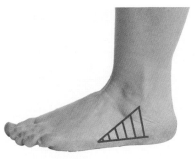

Find the distal end of the metatarsal and cover the triangle as shown in the diagram.

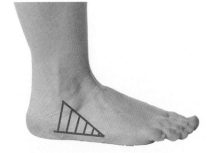

Location on the hands:

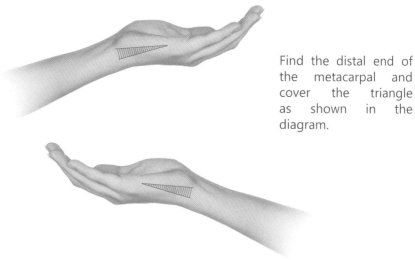

Find the distal end of the metacarpal and cover the triangle as shown in the diagram.

Physiological action

The leg can be separated into two sections: the upper leg, which consists of a single bone (the femur) and attendant muscles that join the pelvis at the hip; and the lower leg, which consists of two bones (tibia and fibula) with attendant muscle that join the foot at the ankle. These are separated by the knee joint. Together, the bones and muscles of the leg are responsible for supporting the body in an upright position, and for all the movements of the leg.

Physical problems or illnesses to be aware of:

When thinking of the leg, it is important to think of all the issues that might affect it and check to see if there are any present now, or whether there have been any problems in this area in the past.

Classic examples would be:

Cramp - the sudden, painful contraction of a muscle, most commonly found in the legs. Although painful, it is not likely to cause any lasting damage.

Dislocation - where the femur has popped out of its socket and the supporting tissues are stretched and/or torn.

Fractured femur, tibia or fibula - where one of the leg bones breaks, usually after a fall.

Leg ulcer - a persistent, open sore, normally found on the lower part of the leg.

Osteogenesis imperfecta - a genetic disorder where the bones break much more easily.

Osteomalacia - where the bones are weak or soft and distort or break easily. This is most often caused by a lack of Vitamin D or calcium. It is also known as rickets in children.

Osteoporosis - a condition that causes bones to become less dense and therefore weaker and more prone to fracture.

Sprains - where one or more of the ligaments is stretched, twisted or torn, usually as a result of excessive force being applied to a joint.

Strains - where muscle fibres stretch or tear. They normally happen when the muscle has been stretched beyond its limits or it has been forced to contract (shorten) too quickly.

Remember that some of the muscles of the leg area can have an effect further up or lower down the body due to their other connections and attachments, so it is worth looking in more depth when faced with a problem in the leg reflex as to whether its connections could come from elsewhere, for example, the changes in muscle use caused by a change in gait (the way one walks).

Remember to state that reflexology is a sensitive therapy that can pick up current issues and past issues – it does not mean there are any major problems and may relate to a physical or an emotional imbalance in the body.

If the leg reflex area is out of balance, consider:

Physical prompts:

- Do they have or have they had any problems with their legs?

- Is there an excess or lack of exercise? *This may be why they are feeling tension here.*

- Do they have or have they had any problems with their hips or knees? *This will affect the flow of energy in this zone – sometimes it can even be blocked energy from higher in the zone e.g. shoulder.*

The knee

Location in body

The knee forms the joint between the upper and the lower leg.

Location on the feet:

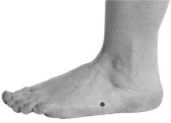

Find the distal end of the 5th metatarsal. Push in and rotate.

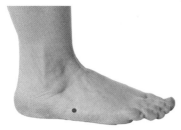

Location on the hands:

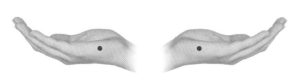

Feel for an indentation on the edge of the hand in Zone 5, halfway between the wrist and the base of the little finger. Push in and rotate.

Physiological action

The knee is the connecting joint between three bones: the femur, the tibia and the fibula, covered over on the anterior side by the patella, which is suspended between tendons. The function of the knee is to provide a hinge joint for flexion and extension of the lower leg. The patella provides extra protection and support to the joint.

Physical problems or illnesses to be aware of:

When thinking of the knee, it is important to think of all the issues that might affect it and check to see if there are any present now, or whether there have been any problems in this area in the past.

Some examples would be:

Arthritis - can take one of two forms. Rheumatoid arthritis is an autoimmune condition where the body's immune system attacks the body. Common symptoms are hot, red, swollen joints and stiffness through the joint. Osteoarthritis is simply wear and tear on the joint that commonly causes pain, stiffness and knobbly or crackly joints.

Bursitis - the inflammation of the bursa (fluid filled sac under the skin usually found around joints), causing pain, inflammation and tenderness. When present in the knee, it is also known as Housemaid's Knee.

A dislocated kneecap - where the patella has come out of its normal position at the front of the knee joint and the surrounding tissues may be torn or overstretched. Dislocation is caused by a sudden change in direction when the leg is planted firmly on the ground.

A fractured knee - where one of the leg bones is broken either on a surface that articulates at the knee, or very close to it. The patella can also be fractured.

Sprains - where one or more of the ligaments is stretched, twisted or torn, usually as a result of excessive force being applied to a joint.

Strains - where muscle fibres stretch or tear. They normally happen when the muscle has been stretched beyond its limits or it has been forced to contract (shorten) too quickly.

Tendonitis - inflammation of a tendon or tendons, causing pain that gets worse on moving the affected area, as well as a grating or crackling sensation, swelling, weakness in the affected area and a lump along the tendon.

Don't forget that some of the muscles around the knee area can have an effect further up or lower down the body due to their other connections and attachments, so it is worth looking in more depth when faced with a problem in the knee reflex as to whether its connections could come from elsewhere; for example, the tension or imbalance could be caused by the changes in muscle use caused by a change in gait (the way one walks).

Remember to state that reflexology is a sensitive therapy that can pick up current issues and past issues – it does not mean there are any major problems and may relate to a physical or an emotional imbalance in the body.

If the knee reflex is out of balance, consider:

Physical prompts:

- Do they have or have they had any problems with their knees?

- Do they do any regular activity which requires bending repeatedly?

- Is there an excess or lack of exercise? *This may be why they are feeling tension here.*

- Do they have or have they had any problems with their hips or legs? *This will affect the flow of energy in this zone – sometimes it can even be blocked energy from higher in the zone e.g. shoulder.*

122

Emotional links: Musculo-skeletal system

If physical issues are present, the emotional involvement may still be important as part of the illness. If none of these are present then it is even more important to consider emotional blocks.

Key area: all areas stand separately; there is no common ground as they are all structural.

Be aware as you listen, not to tell them how you think they should move forward, but instead ask useful questions to allow them to explore the ideas.

Exploring possible emotional reasons for reflexes that are out of balance has to be handled with great sensitivity, and it can be presented purely as one school of thought. It may be that it is not suitable to share this information with your client, but it might help you understand why the reflex is imbalanced. You will need to use careful judgement as to whether to share this information.

The head: *represents the brain area, so consider issues around thinking:*

- What are they spending lots of time thinking about?

- What do they believe?

- Is there something affecting their core beliefs and ideas?

The neck: *represents the connection between head (thoughts) and heart (feelings). People with neck problems often have a disconnect between the two.*

- Do they feel their head and heart are flowing in the same direction?

- What are they not saying that needs to be said?

Alternatively, it can represent an expression:

- Who is being a pain in the neck?

Hard skin on the neck reflex may indicate not wanting to talk about a situation, so it may be sensitive. Consider:

- Do they have something on their mind that they aren't able to express?

The spine: *see page 163 for spine and spinal column, as these would have the same emotional interpretation.*

The shoulder: *reflexes represent shouldering responsibilities .*

- How much responsibility is resting on their shoulders right now?

- Can they think of one way, specifically, that they could make their responsibilities easier to deal with?

- What is it they feel or are told they "should" be doing but don't really want to?

The elbow: *related to with flexibility and direction.*

- Do they need to change direction?

- Are they feeling inflexible emotionally?

- How can they find ways to more easily go with the flow?

The pelvis: *this represents grounding and sense of security to move forward and take the next steps.*
- How secure do they feel about their plans for the future?

- What are they planning?

If there is hard skin here, you can be sure the person is feeling insecure about their plans for the future, so instead consider:
- Is there one thing specifically that they can put in place to allow themselves to feel more secure about putting their plans into action?

The leg: *this is about how you stand, progress and move in life.*
- Are they having problems with where or how they stand in life?

The knee: *all about moving forward.*
- Do they have plans that they can't quite put in motion?

- What can they do to allow themselves to put their plans into action?

The Respiratory System

Introduction

Respiration is breathing in and out. It is a process requiring a specialised system of muscles and tissues which brings the breath of life into the body and expels waste. On inhalation, oxygen is passed through the one cell thick walls of the lung into the blood circulation on the other side; on exhalation, the waste product carbon dioxide is exchanged and carried out of the body. Without it, life is not possible.

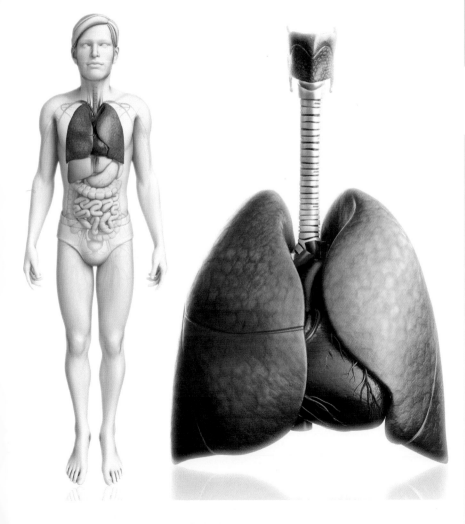

The chest area

Location in body

The chest is the whole of the upper torso under and including the rib cage. This area has layer upon layer of muscles to allow for the movement required for respiration; the ability to receive or inhale (oxygen) and release or exhale (carbon dioxide). This physiological action is required for life.

Location on the feet:

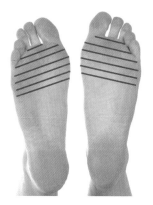

Thumb walk across the feet below the toes and above the diaphragm line.

Location on the hands:

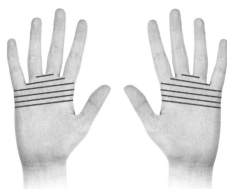

Thumb walk across the hand below the fingers and above the diaphragm line.

Physiological action

Respiration involves the intercostal muscles and the diaphragm. The contraction of the intercostal muscles raises the rib cage, making the width of the chest greater.

The diaphragm

Location in body

This is a large sheet of muscle in a dome shape that separates the chest cavity from the abdominal cavity. Muscle fibres attach to the sternum, the margin of the rib cage, ribs 6-12 and into vertebra T12. There are two added appendages (the left and right crus) that attach to the lumbar vertebrae L1 and L2. There are three openings in the diaphragm, allowing the inferior vena cave and phrenic nerve, the aorta and the oesophagus through.

Location on the feet:

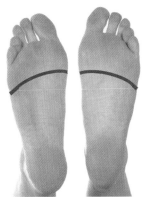

Thumb walk across in a line at the base of the metatarsal bones.

Location on the hands:

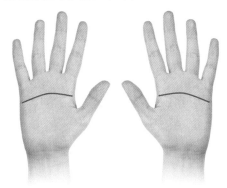

Thumb walk across in a line at the base of the metacarpal bones.

Physiological action

The action of muscles pulls the dome of the diaphragm downwards increasing the available space in the chest cavity; this causes a suction effect that draws air down into the lungs. When the diaphragm relaxes under the recoil due to the elasticity of the muscles, the diaphragm springs back up to position, forcing air out of the lungs. This is called forced expiration. The same muscular action and change in internal pressures are involved with the movement of vomit, faeces and urine.

The lungs

Location in body

The lungs are located in the upper body, under the rib cage. They are large spongy sacks that are involved in the process of respiration.

Bronchi / Bronchioles - The major tube called the trachea brings air into the centre of the lungs through the throat. It branches off into two smaller tubes, one to the left and one to the right, which are called bronchi. The air gets passed down smaller and smaller tubes (bronchioles) until it reaches the main lung tissue. All of these tubes consist of smooth muscle with mucus secreting glands in the wall and are lined with respiratory epithelium which has cilia to remove dust and particles. Each is surrounded by cartilage plates to provide structure and keep the airway open. There is no gas exchange in these tubes.

Location on the feet:

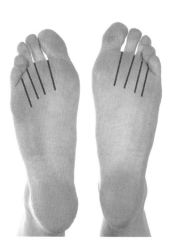

On the plantar aspect of the feet, walk up from the shoulder or diaphragm line to the toes between the metatarsal bones.

Location on the hands:

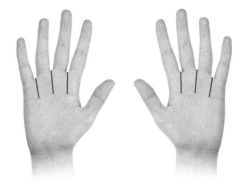

On the palmar aspect of the hand, thumb walk in between each metacarpal bone from the base of the fingers to the diaphragm line.

Physiological action

The main lung tissues consist of alveolar sacs that have walls which are one cell thick. A network of capillaries covers the external and internal lung tissue for exchange of gases from the incoming air to the blood and vice-versa from the blood to the expelled air. On breathing in, oxygen rich air is taken down the trachea into the lungs, where oxygen is transferred through the cells into the blood on the other side.

In contrast, the blood on the inside of the body is carbon dioxide rich (a waste product) as it has travelled all around the body. This carbon dioxide is transferred in the opposite direction from the inner body to the external lung surface and then breathed out. The diaphragm muscle is very involved with the process of breathing in, as when the diaphragm contracts, the chest cavity expands. This causes a vacuum in the chest cavity that brings air into the lungs. When the diaphragm relaxes, the air is expelled.

In short, oxygen (life giving) comes in, whilst carbon dioxide (toxic waste product) goes out.

There is also a 'cleaning' action of the lungs, as the small hairs or cilia that line the tube surfaces remove any particulate matter from the incoming air. These incoming particles can cause irritation or at worst allergic reactions.

The movement of the chest cavity or breathing in and out is under control of the autonomic nervous system. The action happens without conscious thought and can be affected by exercise, stress and reduced oxygen in the air.

Physical problems or illnesses to be aware of:

When thinking of the lungs, it is important to think of all the issues that might affect the lungs and check to see if there are any present now, or if there have been any problems in this area in the past.

Common pathologies would be:

Asthma – the intermittent narrowing of the airways, causing shortness of breath caused by a reaction to an irritant.

Bronchitis – a bacterial or viral infection which often develops opportunistically after a bout of cold or flu. Smokers and others with lung diseases will be more at risk.

Cough – a reflex response to an infection or irritation of the respiratory tract.

Pleurisy – inflammation of the pleura, the external covering of the lungs which separates the lungs from the chest wall.

Pneumonia – inflammation of the lung tissue in one or both lungs as a result of a bacterial or viral infection.

Smoking – this can cause imbalances in the lung reflex but not necessarily in all clients.

Less common pathologies would be:

Emphysema – progressive inflammatory damage to the lungs, resulting in wheezing and shortness of breath. Suffers may also have chronic bronchitis. The two diseases together are known as chronic obstructive pulmonary disease (COPD).

Sarcoidosis – an inflammatory disease leaving small patches of inflammation all over the tissue surface. This is most commonly present in the lungs.

Tuberculosis (TB) – A bacterial infection that most often affects the lungs but can affect other parts of the body.

Whooping cough or Pertussis – an infection of the lining of the airways that causes bouts of coughing.

Remember to state that reflexology is a sensitive therapy that can pick up current issues and past issues – it does not mean there are any major problems and may relate to a physical or an emotional imbalance in the body.

If the chest, diaphragm or lung reflexes are out of balance, consider:

Physical prompts:

- Do they currently have any problems with their lungs or chest?

- Have they had any major problems in the past?

- Are they prone to any lung or breathing problems such as chest infections, asthma etc?

- Do they get any aerobic exercise which allows the lungs to work efficiently? *Be aware, this could be a sign of excessive exercise or too little.*

- Do they hunch over a computer, which may restrict the flow of blood and energy through the lungs?

- Do they have allergies and if so, have they been in contact with that allergen recently?

- Do they smoke?

Emotional links: Respiratory system

If physical issues are present, the emotional involvement may still be important as part of the illness. If none of these are present then it is even more important to consider emotional blocks.

Key area: representing the ability to receive (inhale - oxygen) and release (exhale – carbon dioxide) in the emotional parts of life.

The lungs are all about the breath of life and being able to live in harmony with giving and receiving. Note how deeply or how shallowly your client breathes and understand whether they are embracing all that life has to offer or limiting themselves. Think of the difference in breath between someone having a panic attack and someone stood at the top of a mountain taking the air into their lungs. Lung efficiency can be about feelings of lack of strength and personal power. Breath holding can be about holding onto control. Rapid breathing is holding control when life is moving too fast.

The lungs are like the tree of life. When you look at the lungs, they are like a tree with a trunk, branches and smaller branches (twigs). They need to be strong and flexible like a tree and well rooted in the ground.

When someone is not well rooted in themselves and not grounded and feeling safe, their "tree" can be unstable and the breath of life may be hard to inhale. Inhale - in a helpful way - things that feed their essence (breath of life), with things like new ideas, concepts and life affirming intentions to create good feelings. Lungs also let go of what is not needed or has done its job (waste). It's about being able to receive and let go. Grief can be associated with lung issues too as there may have been something that they are not willing to let go of.

Be aware as you listen, not to tell them how you think they should move forward, but instead ask useful questions to allow them to explore the ideas.

Exploring possible emotional reasons for reflexes that are out of balance has to be handled with great sensitivity, and it can be presented purely as one school of thought. It may be that it is not suitable to share this information with your client, but it might help you understand why the reflex is imbalanced. You will need to use careful judgement as to whether to share this information.

If there are imbalances in the respiratory system, consider:

Emotional prompts

- Do they feel as though they are holding on to any emotions?
- How are they feeling?
- What emotion are they keeping in?
- What emotion might they be keeping to themselves that they don't want others to know?
- To whom do they feel they can't show how they are feeling?
- How long have they been hiding their feelings?
- How do they enjoy and flow with life?
- How much enjoyment do they have in their life?
- Have they been through any major process of grieving in their life? Do they feel they have released all the emotions attached to this time?

The Reproductive System

Introduction

The reproductive system is a system of both internal and external organs which are necessary for sexual reproduction and the creation of new life. It has been claimed that this is the most essential system as without reproduction the human race would die out. However, this system would not function without the sex hormones produced by the endocrine system and the relay of messages through the nervous system to the hypothalamus, which then sends appropriate messages to the pituitary and endocrine system.

The female reproductive system has two main functions; to produce ova and also to protect and nourish the foetus until birth. The function of the male reproductive system is to produce and deliver sperm.

Please note that the ovaries and testes are also part of the reproductive system; you can find these discussed in detail in the endocrine system chapter.

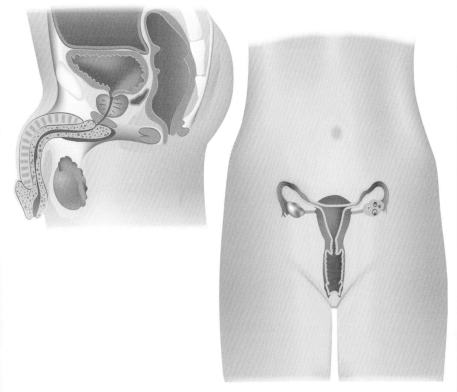

The epididymides

Location in body

The epididymides (pleural) are a single coiled tube found in each scrotum. Each one is approximately 6m long, but as they are fine tubes that are tightly coiled, they form into a 4cm mass around each testis.

The epididymides lie close to the testes in a curved shape covering the whole of the posterior aspect of the testes. They start at the efferent tubule of each testis, pass over the top of the testis and then down the posterior side. Near the base of the testis, they turn 180 degrees to join the Vas deferens.

It is worth knowing that the total maturation and delivery time of sperm is about 3 months, from new cells to ejaculation. This means that any life changes made will take about three months to show in sperm tests.

Location on the feet:

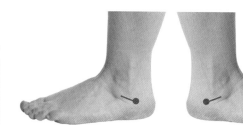

As the epididymis lies mainly posterior to the testis, working the testis reflex will also be working the epididymis. Then use finger or thumb to walk or slide up to the ankle bone where the Vas deferens starts.

Location on the hands:

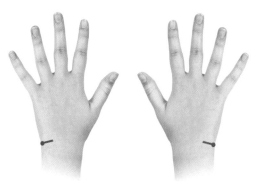

Work the testis reflex and then use finger or thumb to walk or slide up to the wrist bone where the Vas deferens starts.

Physiological action

The epididymis carries sperm from the testis to the Vas deferens. When sperm cells enter the epididymis they are immature, lack motility and are diluted by liquid. The smooth muscle surrounding the epididymis causes slow peristaltic waves, moving the sperm slowly through the 6m tubule over a two week period while the epithelial lining secretes nutrients to help the maturation of the sperm.

Excess liquid is removed by the stereocilia (long cytoplasmic projections that have no motility) which line the tubule to concentrate the sperm and also remove any dead or defective sperm. The sperm can remain in the epididymis for up to two months waiting for ejaculation.

After two months in the epididymis the sperm begin to deteriorate and are then absorbed by the stereocilia. These are then replaced by younger sperm.

During ejaculation the sperm are moved from the lower storage area of the epididymis into the Vas deferens by peristaltic action of the smooth muscle, as sperm are still unable to swim at this stage.

Physical problems or illnesses to be aware of:

When thinking of the epididymides, it is important to think of all the issues that might affect them and check to see if there are any present now, or if there have been any problems in this area in the past.

Epididymitis – the most common cause of acute scrotal pain due to inflammation of the epididymis, causing pain, redness and swelling of the scrotum.

Remember to state that reflexology is a sensitive therapy that can pick up current and past issues – it does not mean there are any major problems and may relate to a physical or an emotional imbalance in the body.

Be particularly aware when discussing reproductive areas, not to cause concern that there may be medical or emotive issues surrounding this area.

If the epididymis reflex is out of balance, consider:

Physical prompts:

- Do they have, or have they ever had any discomfort in the pelvic region?

- Do they sit for long periods with a poor posture, which may be affecting the nerve supply to the pelvis?

N.B. If they are seeing you regarding conception, you can ask if they have had any tests e.g. semen analysis, and ask what the results were.

The Vas deferens

Location in body

The Vas deferens is a tiny muscular tube, approximately 5mm wide and 30cm long, that carries sperm from the epididymis to the ejaculatory ducts in the prostate. There are two Vas deferens; one from the right testis and one from left.

Each Vas deferens joins onto the tail-end of the epididymides in the posterior regions of the scrotum and ascends posterior to the testes through the spermatic cord (a thick walled muscular duct and a cord-like collection of structures which forms a passage from the testis, exiting the scrotum and continuing up through the inguinal canal, into the pelvis).

Once inside the pelvic cavity, the Vas deferens turns toward the bladder, continues around the side of the bladder, passing superior to the ureters and on to the prostate gland. As the Vas deferens approaches the prostate, it widens in a region known as the ampulla, then narrows before joining with the seminal vesicles at the ejaculatory duct inside the prostate.

Location on the feet:

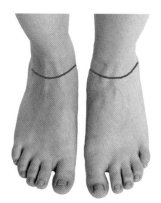

Work from ankle bone to ankle bone using fingers or thumbs. Some therapists like to work in the direction of testis to prostate (lateral to medial) as this is the way sperm travel, while others work in both directions.

Location on the hands:

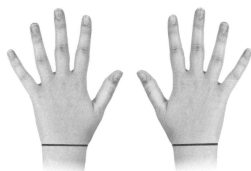

Work from wrist bone to wrist bone using fingers or thumbs. Some therapists like to work in the direction of testis to prostate (lateral to medial) as this is the way sperm travel, while others work in both directions.

Physiological action

During ejaculation, the smooth muscle in the walls of the Vas deferens contracts and relaxes (peristalsis) to move sperm up through the Vas deferens into the ampulla ready for the next ejaculation. Sperm can remain in the ampulla for up to 2-3 months if there is no ejaculation. Old and damaged sperm are absorbed into the body through the epithelial lining of the ampulla.

At the next ejaculation the sperm move from the ampulla towards the urethra by peristalsis, As the sperm pass through the prostate and seminal vesicles, these strucures release secretions that mix with the sperm to form semen (see prostate gland).

Physical problems or illnesses to be aware of:

When thinking of the Vas deferens, it is important to think of all the issues that might affect it and check to see if there are any present now, or if there have been any problems in this area in the past.

Congenital Bilateral Absence of Vas deferens (CBAVD) - obstructed or completely absent Vas deferens; for example, this is common in cystic fibrosis or can result from infections. It can be overcome by surgically collecting sperm from the testicle and using IVF.

Testicular torsion - the testicles twist and strangle the spermatic cord, cutting off the blood supply to the testicles. Torsion can cause atrophy and necrosis if not treated promptly. Signs include scrotal pain, blood in semen, swelling of a testicle and abdominal pain.

Vasectomy – Although not an illness or problem, it is the Vas deferens that is cut in a vasectomy as a form of contraception.

Remember to state that reflexology is a sensitive therapy that can pick up current issues and past issues – it does not mean there are any major problems and may relate to a physical or an emotional imbalance in the body.

Be particularly aware when discussing reproductive areas, not to cause concern that there may be medical or emotive issues surrounding this area.

If the Vas deferens reflex is out of balance, consider:

Physical prompts:

- Do they have, or have they ever had any discomfort in the pelvic region?

- Do they sit for long periods with a poor posture, which may be affecting the nerve supply to the pelvis?

N.B. If they are seeing you regarding conception, you can ask if they have had any tests e.g. semen analysis, and ask what the results were.

The prostate gland

Location in body

The prostate gland is a small muscular gland. It is often said to be the size of a walnut, although it does continue to grow throughout a man's life. It surrounds the urethra just inferior to the bladder, at the point where the urethra exits the bladder in the pelvic cavity. This organ can become enlarged, causing problems.

Location on the feet:

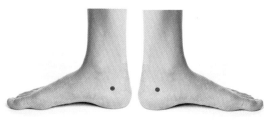

Located on the medial aspect of the foot, half way between the middle maleolus and back of the heel.

Location on the hands:

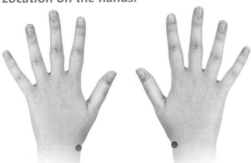

Press into the dip just in front of the wrist bone in Zone 1.

Physiological action

The prostate produces prostatic secretions - a milky white fluid containing sugars, enzymes and an alkaline chemical. This secretion forms approximately 70% of the ejaculate. The sugars provide nutrition for the sperm, the enzymes break down proteins in the semen after ejaculation to allow the sperm to break free from the semen so they are able to fertilize an ovum and the alkaline chemical neutralizes the vaginal secretions to ensure the sperm can survive for longer.

The prostate also contains the ejaculatory duct that releases sperm during ejaculation. This duct opens and the sperm are transmitted from the part of the Vas deferens located in the prostate, and into the urethra by the action of the smooth muscle in the prostate. This contracts to push semen into the urethra and out through the end of the penis.

During urination, urine is released from the bladder and is carried by the urethra down through the penis. The urine normally passes freely through the prostate. However the prostate enlarges slowly throughout a man's lifetime. By the age of approximately 60, this can lead to a restriction or blockage of the urethra, which can cause difficulty in urination or occasionally an inability to pass any urine, which must be seen urgently by a doctor.

Physical problems or illnesses to be aware of:

When thinking of the prostate it is important to think of all the issues that might affect it and check to see if there are any present now, or if there have been any problems in this area in the past.

Benign prostatic hyperplasia – commonly referred to as an obstruction, this generally occurs in older men as the prostate enlarges and can make urination difficult.

139

Prostate cancer – one of the most common cancers affecting older men. If it is localised to the prostate, it is often very slow growing and may never cause problems. For more advanced prostate cancers there are many different treatments including surgical removal, chemotherapy, hormone therapy, and radiotherapy.

Prostatitis - Inflammation of the prostate gland. There are 3 main types: acute prostatitis, chronic bacterial prostatitis and chronic non-bacterial prostatitis. Chronic non-bacterial prostatitis is the most common. Its cause is unknown, but may be linked to problems in the immune system or nervous system, or from an undiscovered viral or bacterial infection.

Remember to state that reflexology is a sensitive therapy that can pick up current issues and past issues – it does not mean there are any major problems and may relate to a physical or an emotional imbalance in the body.

Be particularly aware when discussing reproductive areas, not to cause concern that there may be medical or emotive issues surrounding this area.

140

If the prostate reflex is out of balance, consider:

Physical prompts:

- Do they have any problems urinating? **

- Do they feel the need to go to the toilet frequently? **

- Do they have, or have they ever had any discomfort in the pelvic region?

- Do they sit for long periods with a poor posture, which may be affecting the nerve supply to the pelvis?

*** If the answer to this is yes, they should be referred to a GP. Tell your client to make an appointment to discuss his symptoms. Reassure him that this is probably something minor but is worth checking out.*

The fallopian tubes

Location in body

There are two fallopian tubes, which are about 10cm long and are approximately 0.5 - 1.2 cm in diameter, connecting the ovaries to the uterus. They are located within the pelvic cavity and are connected to the superior lateral edge of the ovaries, travelling across to the superior lateral edge of the uterus.

The fallopian tubes are narrowest and thickest where they border the uterus (called the isthmus); they then begin to get wider as they move towards the ovaries (called ampulla) and then widen further into a funnel shape (infundibulum) as they end at the superior lateral edges of the ovaries. The infundibulum then has finger-like projections (fimbriae) that extend to the surface of the ovaries.

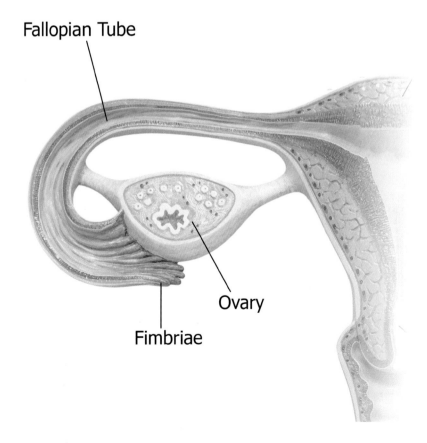

Fallopian Tube

Ovary

Fimbriae

Location on the feet:

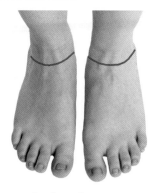

Work from ankle bone to ankle bone using fingers or thumbs. Some therapists like to work in the direction of ovary to uterus (lateral to medial) as this is the way the ovum travels, while others work in both directions.

Location on the hands

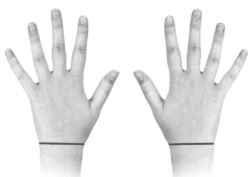

Work from wrist bone to wrist bone using fingers or thumbs. Some therapists like to work in the direction of ovary to uterus (lateral to medial) as this is the way the ovum travels, while others work in both directions.

Physiological action

The fallopian tubes are passageways for the ovum from the ovary to the uterus, and it is here where fertilisation usually occurs. It takes approximately 5 days for the ovum to travel from the ovary to the uterus.

Just prior to ovulation, the fimbriae respond to changing levels of Follicle Stimulating Hormone (FSH) and Luteinizing Hormone (LH) and they begin to slowly contact and relax. This causes a steady sweeping motion over the surface of the ovary ready to catch the ovum as it is released, and will then carry the ovum into the infundibulum. The ovum is then moved into the ampulla and then on towards the isthmus by the beating cilia and peristaltic wave action of the muscular wall.

If sperm enter the uterus, they may enter the fallopian tubes and fertilise an ovum if there is one present. Sperm can stay in the fallopian tubes for up to 7 days, as these provide a safe environment that's conducive to their survival. Some sperm actually bind to the fallopian tube itself, as they can receive direct nourishment from the lining. Ova, however, can only survive for 12-24 hours.

Physical problems or illnesses to be aware of:

When thinking of the fallopian tubes it is important to think of all the issues that might affect them and check to see if there are any present now, or if there have been any problems in this area in the past.

Ectopic Pregnancy - An ectopic pregnancy is where a fertilised egg implants itself outside of the womb, usually in one of the fallopian tubes. Symptoms include abdominal pain and absence of a period. These are usually noticed between 5 and 14 weeks of pregnancy.

Endometriosis - The presence of endometrium cells (the cells that line the interior wall of the uterus) in other parts of the body, such as the fallopian tubes, ovaries, bladder, bowel, vagina or rectum.

Pelvic inflammatory disease - inflammation of the uterus, fallopian tubes, and/or ovaries. If left untreated there can be scar formation. The most common cause is bacterial infection.

Tubal blockage or obstruction – a major cause of female fertility issues. Common causes include pelvic inflammatory disease, endometriosis and abdominal infections such as appendicitis.

143

Remember to state that reflexology is a sensitive therapy that can pick up current issues and past issues – it does not mean there are any major problems and may relate to a physical or an emotional imbalance in the body.

Be particularly aware when discussing reproductive areas, not to cause concern that there may be medical or emotive issues surrounding this area.

If the fallopian tubes reflexes are out of balance, consider:

Physical prompts:

- Do they have very painful periods? *If yes, have they ever seen their GP about these?*

- Do they sit for long periods with a poor posture, which may be affecting the nerve supply to the pelvic area?

- Have they had any problems with their reproductive system in the past?

N.B. If they are seeing you regarding conception, you can ask if they have had any tests e.g. ultra sound scan, laparoscopy etc.

The uterus

Location in body

The uterus is a hollow organ situated in the midline of the pelvis and is where a foetus develops during pregnancy. In a non pregnant state, the uterus is approximately the size of a pear and sits within the pelvic cavity in between the bladder and the rectum. During pregnancy it has the ability to greatly expand out of the pelvic cavity and up to the diaphragm line.

The main cavity is known as the 'body' and superior to this is a domed area known as the fundus; the fallopian tubes join at lateral edges of the fundus. Inferior to the body, the uterus narrows and ends at the cervix, which connects the uterus to the vagina.

Location on the feet:

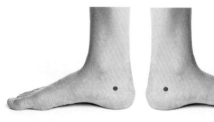

Located on the medial aspect of the foot, half way between the middle malleolus and back of the heel.

Location on the hands:

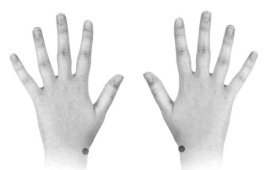

Press into the dip just in front of the wrist bone in Zone 1.

Physiological action

The walls of the uterus have three layers:

1. Perimetrium – the outermost layer that protects the uterus. It is formed from a smooth layer of epithelial cells which secrete a lubricating fluid to prevent friction with other abdominal organs.

2. Myometrium – the centre layer which contains muscle tissue, allowing the uterus to expand during pregnancy and contract during labour.

3. Endometrium – the inner layer of highly vascular connective tissue which has the ability to form a thick lining ready for implantation and formation of a placenta if a zygote (fertilized ovum) implants in the endometrium.

At the time of ovulation, under the influence of oestrogen and progesterone, the endometrium builds a thick layer of endometrial tissue in preparation to receive a zygote. If the ovum is not fertilized, it passes through the uterus and through the cervix. The lack of implantation causes a drop in progesterone and the blood vessels will then begin to deteriorate. The lining is shed and menstruation begins. Many women may experience painful cramps at this time, known as dysmenorrhea, and pain may be felt in the pelvis or lower abdomen but may also be felt in the back. For menstruation to happen, the uterine muscles contract to constrict the blood supply to the endometrium so it will break down and can pass out of the body through the vagina. These contractions and the resulting temporary oxygen deprivation to nearby tissues are responsible for the pain or "cramps" that may be experienced during menstruation.

If the ovum is fertilised, it moves into the uterus and will try to implant into the uterine wall 6-7 days after fertilisation. The cells on the surface of the blastocyst change and become enlarged and sticky (trophoblast cells). The endometrium is also undergoing changes, producing cells which reduce the volume of fluid in the uterus, allowing the embryo to get closer to the walls. The trophoblast cells of the embryo change and start to invade into the surface of the endometrium, resulting in attachment and eventually the setting up of a circulation that becomes the placenta.

During pregnancy, the uterus grows to accommodate the growing foetus. The placenta provides nutrients and oxygen from the mother's blood to the foetus and also removes carbon dioxide and metabolic waste products into the mother's blood for disposal.

At the end of the pregnancy, oxytocin is released from the pituitary, which instructs the myometrium to start contracting, slowly at first then building in strength and frequency, pushing the baby downwards. Once the cervix is fully dilated, the uterine contractions increase dramatically until the baby is born.

Physical problems or illnesses to be aware of:

When thinking of the uterus it is important to think of all the issues that might affect it and check to see if there are any present now, or if there have been any problems in this area in the past.

Adenomyosis - heavy and painful periods as a result of endometrial tissue growing into the myometrium, causing the uterus to be tender and bulky.

Asherman's syndrome - Damage to the basal endometrium resulting in adhesion and/or fibrosis, often as a result of trauma such as surgical termination or a dilation and curettage (D&C).

Dysmenorrhoea - Pain associated with menstruation. In most cases, the pain is a normal part of the menstrual cycle, caused by muscular contractions of the uterine wall. In some cases, dysmenorrhoea is caused by an underlying medical condition such as endometriosis, fibroids, pelvic inflammatory disease, and having an intrauterine contraceptive device fitted.

Endometritis – inflammation of the endometrium, most commonly as a result of infection.

Endometriosis - tissue behaving like the lining of the womb (the endometrium) is found outside the womb.

Fibroids – non-cancerous tumours that grow slowly within the muscular wall of the uterus or around the uterus. They are abnormal growths of muscular and fibrous tissue, occurring singly or in groups. Fibroids can vary in size from the size of a pea to the size of a melon. They are found in about 1 in 4 women of childbearing age and are more common in Afro-Caribbeans. The cause of fibroids is unknown, but they are thought to be linked to the response of the uterus to oestrogen. This link is likely to be the reason why fibroids tend to grow at times of high oestrogen level and shrink after the menopause when the oestrogen level falls. The likelihood of fibroids increases with obesity.

Prolapse - occurs when the ligaments supporting the uterus become weak and cannot hold the uterus in place, so it slips down from its normal position into the vagina. Can be a result of a traumatic birth.

Remember to state that reflexology is a sensitive therapy that can pick up current issues and past issues – it does not mean there are any major problems and may relate to a physical or an emotional imbalance in the body.

Be particularly aware when discussing reproductive areas, not to cause concern that there may be medical or emotive issues surrounding this area.

If the uterus reflex is out of balance, consider:

Physical prompts:

- How are their periods? Would they describe them as particularly heavy or painful?

- Do they get any pain or bloating in their abdomen? *If yes, have they ever seen their GP about this?*

- Do they currently have their period?

- Do they sit for long periods with a poor posture, which may be affecting the nerve supply to the pelvic area?

N.B. If they are seeing you regarding conception, you can ask if they have had any tests e.g. ultra sound scan, laparoscopy etc.

The cervix

Location in body

The cervix is the lower part of the uterus and is approximately 2 - 3 cm long. It is round in shape and lies between the bladder and the rectum. It is divided into 3 regions:

1. Internal os - superior opening from the uterus into the cervical canal.

2. Cervical canal - hollow orifice through the cervix that connects the uterine cavity to the vagina.

3. External os - inferior opening from the cervical canal to the vagina. This is surrounded by external tissue of the cervix which protrudes slightly into the vagina.

Location on the feet:

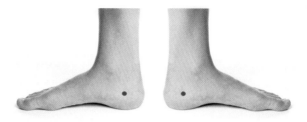

The cervix reflex is located on the medial aspect, half way between the middle of the malleolus and the back of the heel. Place your thumb on this reflex and rock your thumb down towards the bladder reflex. You will feel the ridge of the calcaneous bone which is the location of the cervix reflex.

N.B. THIS MUST NOT BE WORKED IN PREGNANCY.

Location on the hands:

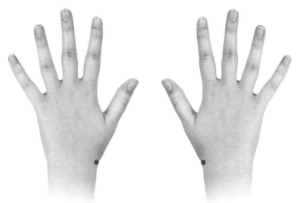

The cervix reflex is located in the dip just in front of the wrist bone in the zone 1, where the wrist articulates. Rest your thumb on this reflex and push towards the base of the scaphoid bone (your thumb moves slightly towards the palmer aspect and you will feel the edge of the scaphoid at the base of the thumb).

N.B. THIS MUST NOT BE WORKED IN PREGNANCY.

Physiological action

The cervix acts as a passageway from the uterine cavity to the vagina and plays vital roles in the control of movement into and out of the uterus, as well as protecting the foetus during pregnancy and during childbirth.

The tissues of the cervix are a continuation of the uterine tissues (3 layers) although the myometrium (middle muscular layer) is thinner than in the uterus as it is only required to control the opening of the cervix.

The cervix controls what substances can pass into and out of the uterus. The endometrium contains epithelial cells that produce cervical mucus, which fills the cervical canal and forms a mucous plug, helping to block the flow of material between the uterus and the vagina. As ovulation approaches, the cervical mucous becomes thinner and more copious (as a result of high oestrogen levels), which allows the passage of sperm into the uterus ready for fertilisation. At this time, the mucous becomes more alkaline and therefore more hospitable for sperm and a better medium for the sperm to journey in. During pregnancy, this mucous plug seals the uterus to protect it from external pathogens.

If the ovum passes unfertilized, menstruation will begin; both blood and endometrial tissue pass through the cervix and then the vagina.

During childbirth, the cervix is required to dilate to allow the foetus to pass into the birth canal. This process can start several days before formal labour starts, with the cervix becoming shorter and softer and starting to slowly dilate. During formal labour the cervix must dilate to 10cm to allow the head and then the body of the foetus to descend. The myometrium is responsible for the opening up of the cervix, which also becomes shorter as it opens up (effacement).

Physical problems or illnesses to be aware of:

When thinking of the cervix it is important to think of all the issues that might affect it and check to see if there are any present now, or if there have been any problems in this area in the past.

Cervical cancer - an uncommon type of cancer that develops in a woman's cervix. The NHS provide screening programmes as with early detection this is often curable.

Cervicitis - inflammation of the cervix, usually as a result of infection.

Cervical polyps - benign growths in the cervical canal.

Human papillomaviruses (HPVs) - a group of over 40 viruses that infect genital epithelial cells including the cervix; most are sexually transmitted and can cause warts.

Incompetent cervix - a pregnant woman's cervix begins to dilate and thin before her pregnancy has reached term, which may cause miscarriage or pre-term labour.

Remember to state that reflexology is a sensitive therapy that can pick up current issues and past issues – it does not mean there are any major problems and may relate to a physical or an emotional imbalance in the body.

Be particularly aware when discussing reproductive areas, not to cause concern that there may be medical or emotive issues surrounding this area.

If the cervix reflex is out of balance, consider:

Physical prompts:

150

- Have they been aware of any problems with their cervix before? *This could be during pregnancy or not.*

Be aware that the cervix is connected to the vagina, and sometimes if thrush, vaginal dryness etc. has been an issue, the cervix may show up as well.

The vagina

Location in body

The vagina is an elastic, muscular tube that connects the uterus to the vulva and exterior body. It is located in the pelvic girdle and lies in between the bladder and the rectum. It is approximately 7cm long and 2cm wide. However, during sexual intercourse and childbirth it can become significantly wider and longer.

Location in the feet:

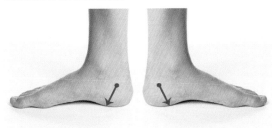

From the uterus and cervix reflex, push down or thumb walk towards the bladder reflex.

Location on the hands:

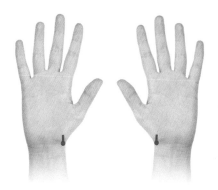

From the uterus and cervix reflex, push down or thumb walk towards the bladder reflex.

Physiological action

During sexual intercourse, the vagina functions as the vessel for the penis and acts as a passageway for sperm through to the cervix, uterus and fallopian tubes. The elastic structure of the vagina allows it to stretch in both length and diameter to accommodate the penis.

Watery secretions (vaginal transudation) produced by the vaginal epithelium lubricate the vagina and have an acidic pH to prevent the growth of bacteria and yeast. The acidic pH also makes the vagina an inhospitable environment for sperm, which is why males produce alkaline seminal fluid to neutralize the acid, adding to the effect of the alkaline cervical secretions around ovulation to improve the survival of sperm. Vaginal secretions decline at menopause as oestrogen reduces.

During childbirth, the vagina acts as the birth canal from the uterus and out of the mother's body into the real world. Once again, the vagina's elasticity allows it to greatly increase its diameter to accommodate the baby.

Finally, the vagina provides a passageway for menstrual flow from the uterus to exit the body during menstruation.

Physical problems or illnesses to be aware of:

When thinking of the vagina it is important to think of all the issues that might affect it and check to see if there are any present now, or if there have been any problems in this area in the past.

Genital herpes - a genital infection caused by the herpes simplex virus. Lesions may appear on or near the pubis, clitoris or other parts of the vagina or vulva.

Vaginal infections - the three most common types are:

- Yeast infections (Candida vulvovaginitis).
- Bacterial infections (bacterial vaginosis).
- Parasitic infections (trichomoniasis).

Vaginitis - a general term for inflammation of the vagina. This is a common condition often caused by infections. It may be but is not always sexually transmitted.

Vaginismus - an involuntary tightening of the vagina muscles during vaginal penetration caused by either a conditioned reflex or a medical condition in the area.

152

Remember to state that reflexology is a sensitive therapy that can pick up current issues and past issues – it does not mean there are any major problems and may relate to a physical or an emotional imbalance in the body.

Be particularly aware when discussing reproductive areas, not to cause concern that there may be medical or emotive issues surrounding this area.

If the vagina reflex is out of balance, consider:

Physical prompts:

- Do they feel they have any problems in this area? *They may have had thrush, or may have some vaginal dryness – this is more common in the menopause.*

Note: these are not reflexes that all therapists include in their treatments. If you do include these you will need to feel confident to handle these conversations as they are of a personal nature. You may wish to wait until the client has had a couple of treatments and is more comfortable with you.

Emotional links: Reproductive system

If physical issues are present, the emotional involvement may still be important as part of the illness. If none of these are present then it is even more important to consider emotional blocks.

Key areas: grounding (links to base chakra) and replication of self. This also can include how secure you are feeling.

Some reproductive and pelvic issues relate to when people are finding it hard or painful to be truly themselves, grounded or happy with themselves. Grounding energy can allow us to feel safe and secure; it connects the head to the ground or base. Many people are energetically 'in their heads' and need to reconnect with the ground or base. The base energy allows us to be rooted, grounded and who we truly are, and allows us to know how to live practically whilst feeling safe and secure.

Be aware as you listen, not to tell them how you think they should move forward, but instead ask useful questions to allow them to explore the ideas.

Exploring possible emotional reasons for reflexes that are out of balance has to be handled with great sensitivity, and it can be presented purely as one school of thought. It may be that it is not suitable to share this information with your client, but it might help you understand why the reflex is imbalanced. You will need to use careful judgement as to whether to share this information.

The reproductive system

Emotional prompts

- If they could truly be themselves, here on Earth, who would they be? How would they be living, experiencing life?

- What changes do they need to make or could they make to be more of who they really are?

- How secure or insecure are they feeling about the future?

- What one thing specifically could they do to help themselves to feel more secure and allow them to move forward to take the next steps?

The Nervous System

Introduction

The nervous system as a whole is the central nervous system together with the peripheral nervous system.

The central nervous system (CNS) comprises the brain and spinal cord. The nerves that come to and from the spinal cord and into the body are the peripheral nervous system (PNS). Both consist of white and grey matter to greater and lesser extents, the white matter being made up of axons which conduct electrical impulses and oligodendrocytes which support and insulate axons, while the grey matter is comprised of neurones.

As a structure, the nervous system co-ordinates and integrates information which then influences activities. It receives and translates sensory information and produces movement.

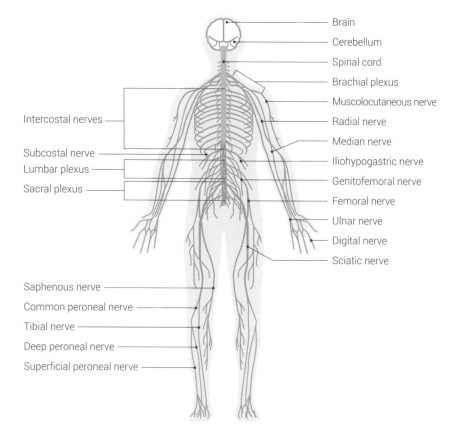

Brain

Cerebellum

Spinal cord

Brachial plexus

Muscolocutaneous nerve

Intercostal nerves

Radial nerve

Median nerve

Subcostal nerve

Iliohypogastric nerve

Lumbar plexus

Genitofemoral nerve

Sacral plexus

Femoral nerve

Ulnar nerve

Digital nerve

Sciatic nerve

Saphenous nerve

Common peroneal nerve

Tibial nerve

Deep peroneal nerve

Superficial peroneal nerve

The Central Nervous System (CNS)

This comprises the brain and spinal cord.

The Brain

This is the major processing unit of the CNS. It is protected by the meninges and encased in the skull. It is comprised of many parts which communicate with the sensory and motor aspects of the body.

Location on the feet:

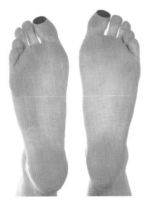

Rub over the top of the big toe with the thumb or knuckle.

Location on the hands:

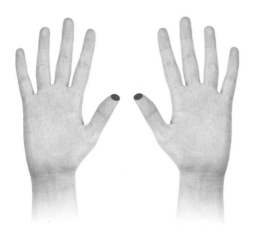

Rub over the top of the thumb with the knuckle of your index finger or thumb.

Brain part	Structure	Physiological action
Medulla	Extension of the spinal cord.	Regulates blood pressure and breathing. Involved in balance, taste, hearing and controls the face and neck muscles.
Pons	Transmits information from cerebellum to cortex.	Breathing, sleep and taste.
Midbrain	Links the motor system, the cerebellum, the basal ganglia and both cerebral hemispheres.	Visual and auditory systems including automatic eye movements.
Brain stem	Entry and exit to the brain for the most important nerve pathways.	Motor and autonomic control of face and neck via the cranial nerves; of the organs via the vagus nerve, also of the heart, blood vessels and pupils.
Cerebellum	Consists of several dividing fissures and lobes, but has more neurones than any other part of the brain.	Posture and co-ordination of the eyes, limbs and head. The learning of new movements and language; also cognition.
Diencephalon which contains	Receives signals from incoming PNS and optic nerve.	Wakefulness and consciousness.
Thalamus	Involved in the sorting of incoming information. Includes Suprachiasmatic nucleus (SCN).	Controls circadian rhythms.
Hypothalamus	Links nervous system to the endocrine system via the pituitary gland (hypophysis).	Primitive emotions, hunger, thirst and maternal bonding via the pituitary hormones. Motivation.

Brain part	Structure	Physiological action
Cerebrum consisting of: 2 cerebral hemispheres, corpus callosum, hippocampus, amygdala, basal ganglion and other nerve fibres.	Largest part of brain.	Planning and carrying out everyday tasks. Co-ordination of voluntary movement, memories, perception and communication of tasks.

The spinal cord

The spinal cord consists mainly of neural tissue enclosed by meninges and protected by the bones of the vertebrae. It extends from the medulla oblongata in the brain, passing through a hole in the skull called the foramen magnum and becomes the spinal column, which finishes at around the second lumbar vertebra. The spinal process passes information to the brain through thalamus and cortex.

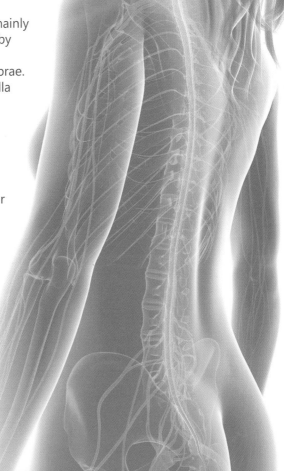

Location on the feet:

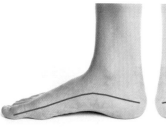

The spinal cord is inside the vertebrae of the spine. Work down the inside of the foot on the bone. Rub across the spine at right angles to work spinal nerves.

Location on the hands:

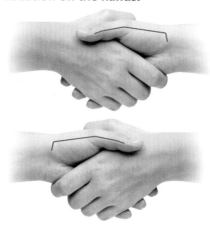

Shake hands with your client; rotate the hand so you can walk from the tip of the thumb to the base of the hand along the bone. Rub across the spine at right angles to work spinal nerves.

Physiological action

The spinal cord has 31 spinal nerves that produce the efferent (outgoing) motor signals and receive the afferent (incoming) sensory signals. These control voluntary and involuntary muscle movement and the perception of the senses.

There are also an additional 10 of the 12 nerves that are part of the PNS but synapse directly on to the CNS. These are the cranial nerves and they provide information from the face, trapezius muscle and cervical spinal nerves. They include the optic and olfactory nerves which means the information gained by the skin in the nose has a direct connection with the brain. This is important for knowing about the environment, for administration of drugs and potentially for aromatherapy too.

Remember to state that reflexology is a sensitive therapy that can pick up current issues and past issues – it does not mean there are any major problems and may relate to a physical or an emotional imbalance in the body.

If the spinal cord or spinal nerve reflexes are out of balance, consider:

Physical prompts:

- Are they very anxious or stressed?
- Do they suffer from the sensation of pins and needles anywhere in the body?
- Do they have any feelings of numbness anywhere in the body?

The Peripheral Nervous System (PNS)

This consists of the nerves and nerve clusters (ganglia) outside of the brain and spinal cord. It relays information and messages between the brain and the extremities. The main differences between the CNS and the PNS are those of protection and insulation. Because the CNS is enclosed within the skull and vertebrae, it is protected from physical damage. There is also the blood brain barrier which protects the CNS from toxins. The PNS does not have these protective layers and so is more open to toxins and mechanical damage. When it comes to insulation, because the nerves in the PNS have to conduct electrical stimuli much further, they have to be better insulated. The insulation comes from myelin produced by the Schwann cells. In the CNS the myelin comes from one oligodendrocyte for many neurones.

Physiological actions

The PNS is split into two parts: the autonomic nervous systems (ANS) and the somatic or voluntary nervous system.

The Autonomic Nervous System (ANS)

This controls involuntary movement below the level of consciousness such as rate of breathing, pupil reaction or heart rate. The ANS is in turn separated into three main nervous system branches.

- Sympathetic – stimulates the body's 'fight or flight' response (opposite to parasympathetic). Promotes fast, responsive actions.
- Parasympathetic – stimulates 'rest and digest' or 'feed and breed' actions (opposite to sympathetic). Provides a slower, dampening action.
- Enteric – can operate autonomously and oversees the function of the gastrointestinal system.

These systems may operate alone or in collaboration with other systems. The parasympathetic and sympathetic operate in opposition to one another; where one actions a physiological response, the other inhibits it.

The Somatic or Voluntary Nervous System

This is responsible for the voluntary control of body movements via the skeletal muscles. It comprises afferent nerves which relay sensations to the CNS and efferent nerves which stimulate muscle contractions.

Location on hands and feet

The peripheral nervous system is extensive and present all over the body; therefore, any efflurage or all over stroking will be relaxing the nervous system.

Physical problems or illnesses to be aware of:

When thinking of the nervous system, it is important to think of all the issues that might affect it and check to see if there are any present now, or whether there have been any problems in this area in the past.

Classic examples would be:

Stress - the firing of alert signals in the amygdala in the brain promotes an imbalance of the hormonal system that leads to the 'fight or flight' response, causing changes in the nervous and muscular systems.

160

Alzheimer's disease - A progressive deterioration in mental ability due to degeneration of brain tissue. It is the most common cause of dementia (the progressive loss of mental abilities).

Epilepsy - Seizures are symptomatic of abnormal electrical activity in the brain. There are 3 main types:

> 1. Symptomatic - when there is a known cause (e.g. brain injury, drug or alcohol abuse, meningitis, stroke and brain tumour).
>
> 2. Idiopathic – when there is no known cause.
>
> 3. Cryptogenic - when there is no known cause but there is evidence (such as learning disorders) to suggest that it may be due to brain damage.

Meningitis - Inflammation of the meninges (the membranes that cover the brain and spinal cord).

Migraine - Intense headache. There are two types: common migraine, which is a severe headache with no warning symptoms, and classical migraine, in which the headache is experienced after warning symptoms (collectively known as the "aura") such as visual disturbances, anxiety, mood swings, changes in energy levels, co-ordination problems, speech difficulties, muscular stiffness or tingling in the neck and shoulders, and an altered sense of taste and smell.

Myalgic encephalomyelitis - Abbreviated to M.E., it literally means muscle pain and inflammation of the brain and spinal cord.

Motor Neurone Disease - Progressive degeneration of the nerves in the brain and spinal cord that control muscular activity.

Muscular Dystrophy - A group of genetic conditions in which muscles become weak and wasted.

Multiple Sclerosis (MS) - A progressive disease of the brain and spinal cord in which the insulating sheaths of the nerves break up and patches of excessive connective tissue form.

Neuralgia - Literally means nerve (neur-) pain (-algia). There are 2 main types: trigeminal neuralgia, which is a sudden and severe nerve pain that affects the face for just a few minutes, and postherpetic neuralgia, which is a constant and severe nerve pain brought on by shingles.

Parkinson's Disease - A progressive brain disorder characterized by tremors, rigidity and impairment of voluntary movement.

Shingles - An viral infection of a nerve and the area of skin that follows its path.

Stroke - Damage to a part of the brain caused by an interruption in its blood supply.

Remember to state that reflexology is a sensitive therapy that can pick up current issues and past issues – it does not mean there are any major problems and may relate to a physical or an emotional imbalance in the body.

If the nervous system is out of balance, consider:

Physical prompts:

- Do they consider themselves to be an anxious person?

- Are they under high levels of stress?

- Do they think they have a high tolerance for stress?

- Do they need to exercise and feel unwell if they don't? *This can indicate a high fight or flight response stimulation, because the arms and legs are full of pumping blood which has to be released by exercise and therefore may be an indicator of high stress levels.*

- Do they suffer from headaches of any sort?

- Do they have, or have they had in the past, any diagnosed illnesses relating to their nervous system?

Emotional links: Nervous system

If physical issues are present, the emotional involvement may still be important as part of the illness. If none of these are present then it is even more important to consider emotional blocks.

Key area: a central system which is central to us as human beings; our life and living, including core beliefs, ideas, and self-esteem.

When anything or anyone gets on our nerves, it can affect our nerves, nervousness or how we respond and react to things.

- Is there something or someone that is getting on their nerves at the moment?

The CNS is our alarm and alert system, so if we are always alert and looking for problems, the CNS will find them around every corner! Our nervous system is constantly responding to our emotions and perception of life. The body responds to whatever our brain is saying to us and so every thought will have a direct effect on the body. The quality of the thoughts can directly affect the physical body.

Nervous system issues can actually stem back to a past disturbance when there was a time of fear – when we were truly nervous and the tremor or potential trigger is still resting in the system. What we think about directly affects our moods, emotions and how our body responds. If our mind is highly attuned to be aware of constant threats (real or perceived), the person can be living on red alert when in actual fact life is fine. The previous big emotional situation or trauma is actually in the past and whilst it is not happening in the current time, the effects may be being brought forward. Being aware of the current time is a great circuit breaker – it's not happening now – it's a past experience that is triggering; however, it's not real, even though it feels real.

Be aware as you listen, not to tell them how you think they should move forward, but instead ask useful questions to allow them to explore the ideas.

Exploring possible emotional reasons for reflexes that are out of balance has to be handled with great sensitivity, and it can be presented purely as one school of thought. It may be that it is not suitable to share this information with your client, but it might help you understand why the reflex is imbalanced. You will need to use careful judgement as to whether to share this information.

Reflexologists can help people with CNS issues by helping them to focus on the 'now'; by helping them to feel confident in themselves to notice and be grateful for what is right (rather than what might be wrong).

The brain *represents core beliefs, ideas and also self-esteem. If someone is constantly knocking your beliefs, your self-esteem will suffer. If you find your client fixates about one specific belief, you might consider:*

- Is there something or someone that is getting on their nerves at the moment?

- Have they had a traumatic or emotional episode in the past? If so, do they think that how they feel now might be related to that time?

- Do they need to let go of past trauma? *This may require extra help from other health professionals*

- Saying "That's one solution; can you think of any other solutions?"

The spine: *our core and central support – it relates to support received but also how we stand up to things, people and situations.*

- Are they getting enough support?

- Where would they like more support in their life right now?

- Who might they need to stand up to in their life?

Lower spine issues relate to the biggest core worry that is often at the root of things for most people in the western world, and can represent a lack of financial support.

- Do they feel unsupported, specifically in the financial area of their life?

The Sensory System

Introduction

Humans are not isolated beings - whilst much of this book has been written about the internal processes of the body, now we move to our interaction with the outside world. Without the sensory system, we would not be able to appreciate the sights, sounds, smells and tastes of the outside world, nor to feel its different textures. Equally, we would not be able to perceive potential dangers; we could not spot flames or something falling towards us; we could not taste the bitterness of poisonous food; we could not smell if food was rancid, feel an earthquake or hear an alarm or the skid of car brakes. The senses offer the body information about the world around us which enables us to function safely and successfully within our environment.

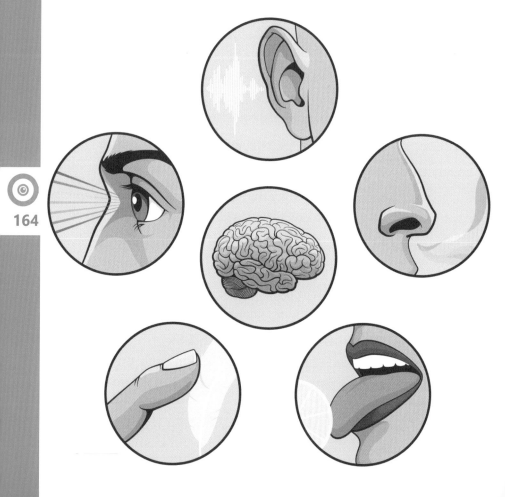

The eyes

Location in body

The eyes are situated in the upper left and upper right quadrants of the face.

Location on the feet:

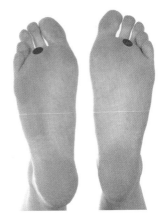

Work down into the top edge of the foot from the webbing between toes 2 and 3.

Location on the hands:

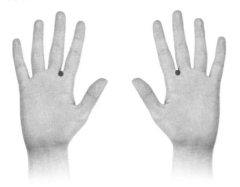

Work down into the top edge of the palm from the webbing between the index and middle fingers.

Physiological action

The eye is a spherical structure which consists of several parts that do different jobs. It is easiest to think of the action of each of the parts by imagining the passage of light through the eye. The first surface the light touches is the conjunctiva, a clear, protective layer over the front of the eye. Next, it hits the cornea, which is a thicker clear layer at the front of the eye that focuses the light in a similar manner to a camera lens. From here it passes through the pupil, a hole that determines how much light is let into the eye, whose size is controlled by the action of the iris (the coloured part that is made up of muscular fibres that contract and expand to control the size of the pupil). The lens then focuses the light more, adjusted by the muscles around it to be either thick and round or thin and flat depending on how close the object is that the eye is looking at. Passing through the vitreous body (a clear, jelly-like substance that maintains the shape of the eye), the light finally arrives at the retina, a layer of photosensitive cells that interpret the image. The retina is made up of two types of cell: rods (that can only process in black and white) and cones (that process in colour). The resulting signal is then transferred through to the optic nerve at the posterior of the eye, which takes the signal to the brain for interpretation into a complete image. The retina is nourished by the choroid, which is a layer of blood vessels running beneath it. The rest of the eye is shaped by the sclera, which forms the 'white' of the eye, encircling the back of the eye and the beginning of the optic nerve. Muscles also attach to the sclera to enable the eye to move in different directions. The eyelids form a further protective layer around the eye, which also carry moisture from the tear ducts across the surface of the eye when one blinks.

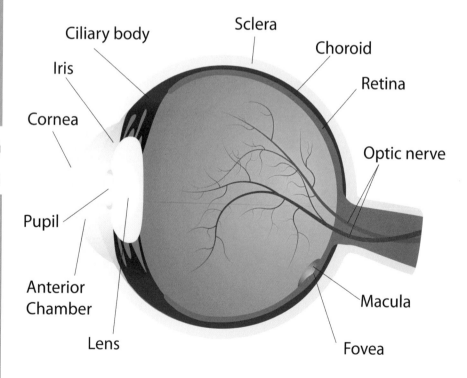

Physical problems or illnesses to be aware of:

When thinking of the eyes, it is important to think of all the issues that might affect the eyes and check to see if there are any present now, or whether there have been any problems with this area in the past.

Common pathologies would be:

Astigmatism - a defect of the eye where the cornea or lens is not perfectly curved, causing the light to not focus properly on the retina, leading to blurry vision. Most people who wear glasses or contact lenses have some form of astigmatism.

Cataracts - the clouding of the lens in the eye, which leads to blurred or distorted vision. They usually develop in both eyes, although one is usually more badly affected than the other. Although they can be due to a congenital condition, cataracts are more common in those over the age of 75.

Conjunctivitis - an infection or inflammation of the conjunctiva. It is also known as pink-eye.

Corneal abrasion - where there is a scratch on the cornea.

Corneal ulcer - a deep erosion of the cornea, caused by injury and/or infection. Contact lens wearers are at greater risk.

Glaucoma - abnormally high pressure in the fluid inside the eye, caused by a blockage where it would normally flow out of the eye. It is more common in those over the age of 60 and runs in families.

A stye - a small, painful red lump on the eyelid. It is usually caused by bacterial infection.

Remember to state that reflexology is a sensitive therapy that can pick up current issues and past issues – it does not mean there are any major problems and may relate to a physical or an emotional imbalance in the body.

If the eye reflexes are out of balance, consider:

Physical prompts:

- Do they have or have they had any problems with their eyes?

- Do they work for long periods on a computer or other types of screens?

- Do they wear glasses and if so, have they had an eye test recently?

- Do they have any sinus problems at the moment?

- Do they suffer from hay fever or itchy eyes?

The ears

Location in body

The ears are situated on the side of the head, approximately halfway between the top of the head and the bottom of the jaw.

Location on the feet:

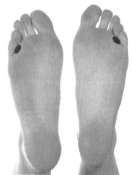

Work down into the top edge of the foot from the webbing between toes 4 and 5.

Location on the hands:

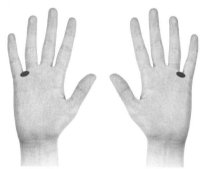

Work down into the top edge of the palm from the webbing between the ring finger and the little finger.

Physiological action

The ear consists of three main parts: the outer ear, the middle ear and the inner ear. The outer ear comprises the pinna (the part you can see) and the auditory canal (also known as the external acoustic meatus). The pinna collects and focuses the sound wave; the auditory canal carries the sound wave through to the middle ear, focusing it further until it meets the eardrum (also known as the tympanic membrane).

The middle ear consists of the eardrum (tympanic membrane) and three tiny bones (ossicles). When the sound wave hits the eardrum, it causes the eardrum to vibrate. The ossicles consist of malleus, incus and stapes (hammer, anvil and stirrup bones), which transfer and amplify the vibration from the eardrum to the inner ear as a physical vibration.

The inner ear consists of a membrane called the oval window, as well as the semi-circular canals, the cochlea and the cochlear nerve. The oval window transfers the vibrations from the ossicles to the cochlea. The cochlea transfers the physical sound vibrations into electric nerve impulses, which are then passed to the brain for interpretation via the cochlear nerve. The semi-circular canals (also known as the labyrinths) are responsible for helping the body to maintain balance.

Physical problems or illnesses to be aware of:

When thinking of the ears, it is important to think of all the issues that might affect the ears and check to see if there are any present now, or whether there have been any problems in this area in the past.

Common pathologies would be:

Cerumen (ear wax) impaction - where ear wax blocks the ear canal and adheres to the eardrum, which may impair hearing.

Deafness - the partial or total loss of hearing, which may be inherited or caused by injury, disease or age.

Earache - pain in the ear. This can be caused by a variety of other conditions or by blockages, including mucus build-up after a cold or toothache.

169

Glue ear - most commonly found in children, where fluid builds up in the middle ear.

Labyrinthitis - a bacterial or viral infection of the semi-circular canals causing balance problems and nausea.

Meniere's disease - a condition where the inner ear on one side of the head malfunctions, which may cause vertigo, tinnitus, hearing loss and/or pain as symptoms.

Ruptured eardrum - where a small hole is torn in the eardrum, usually caused by very loud noises, changes in air pressure, infection or foreign objects.

Tinnitus - the false perception of sounds, usually ringing, buzzing or whistling, originating from one or both ears. The volume perceived may vary; however, these sounds are not audible to anyone except the person with tinnitus.

Vertigo - a false sensation of movement, often combined with nausea and vomiting, making it difficult, if not impossible, to stand up or walk.

Remember to state that reflexology is a sensitive therapy that can pick up current issues and past issues – it does not mean there are any major problems and may relate to a physical or an emotional imbalance in the body.

If the ear reflexes are out of balance, consider:

Physical prompts:

- Do they have or have they had any problems with their ears?

- Do they ever get a feeling of dizziness?

- Do their ears feel as if they are blocked?

- Do they work in a loud environment or listen to loud music?

The nose

Location in body

The nose is situated on the central part of the face, with the nasal cavity extending back into the skull. The olfactory nerve delivers information directly into the brain, which is why inhalation can be used as an effective drug delivery system and why aromatherapy works so well.

Location on the feet:

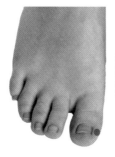
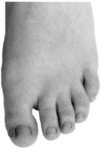

Massage in tiny circles just beneath the middle of the nail line on the big toe.

Location on the hands:

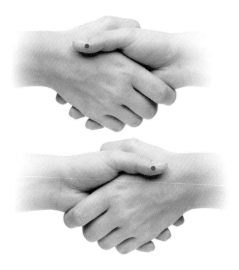

Massage in tiny circles just beneath the middle of the nail line on the thumb.

Physiological action

The nose can be separated into two sections; the external nose and the nasal cavity, both of which are separated by the septum.

The external nose consists of the nasal bone, part of the cheekbones, the nasal part of the frontal bone and plates of hyaline cartilage, all covered over with skin. The arrangement of these components forms the nostrils which allow air in through a hair-lined cavity which filters solid debris from the air we breathe in.

After this, the air moves into the nasal cavity, where it mingles with the mucous lining, producing chemicals for the olfactory nerves to detect. The olfactory nerves carry the signal to the brain, which then interprets it as a particular smell. The rest of the air in the cavity is warmed and moistened some more, passing down to the trachea and on to the lungs for gaseous exchange. The sinuses also take part in this by warming and moistening air that is drawn into them. Another function of the nasal cavity is to act as a resonance box for the voice, in order to make it louder.

Physical problems or illnesses to be aware of:

When thinking of the nose, it is important to think of all the issues that might affect the nose and check to see if there are any present now, or whether there have been any problems with this area in the past.

Common pathologies would be:

Allergic rhinitis - irritation of the inside of the nose by breathing in an allergen (e.g. pollen for those with hay fever), commonly identified by itching, sneezing and a blocked or runny nose.

Nasal polyps - abnormal tissue growths inside the nasal passages or the sinuses.

Nosebleed (epistaxis) - bleeding from the nose, usually caused by injury or the membranes of the nose becoming dry and cracked due to environmental factors.

Sinusitis - the lining of the sinuses becoming inflamed, usually caused by a viral infection.

Snoring - when breathing becomes noisy during sleep, caused by the soft tissues at the back of the nose, mouth and throat vibrating as the person breathes.

Remember to state that reflexology is a sensitive therapy that can pick up current issues and past issues – it does not mean there are any major problems and may relate to a physical or an emotional imbalance in the body.

If the nose reflex is out of balance, consider:

Physical prompts:

- Do they have or have they had any problems with their nose, such as itchiness, sneezing, feeling of a blocked nose, or nose bleeds?

- Are they prone to getting blocked sinuses?

- Do they suffer from allergies or hay fever?

The mouth (see also the mouth in the digestive system section on page 71)

Location in body

The mouth is situated in the centre of the lower part of the face.

Location on the feet:

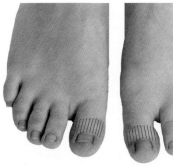

Work on the big toe, from below the nail down to first joint.

Location on the hands:

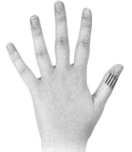
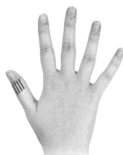

Work on the thumb, from below the nail down to first joint

Physiological action

The mouth can be separated into three main functions (taste, chewing action and formation of sound) and one secondary function (inhalation and exhalation).

For taste, the tongue (situated in the medial base of the mouth) has millions of sensory receptors on its surface. These nerve cells work in a similar manner to those situated in the nasal cavity; food is mixed with liquid (saliva) in the mouth, and the resultant chemical mixture causes the nerve cells in the tongue to fire off signals to the brain for interpretation.

The chewing action involves the lips and cheeks to keep the food in the mouth; the teeth to grind the food into small pieces, thus increasing surface area of food exposed to the chemicals used for digestion; and the muscular action of the tongue to position the food for the teeth and for swallowing.

For inhalation and exhalation, the mouth is only normally used if the nose is blocked. The mouth cavity warms and moistens the air, which then passes through to the trachea and through to the lungs for gaseous exchange to take place.

Physical problems or illnesses to be aware of:

When thinking of the mouth, it is important to think of all the issues that might affect the mouth and check to see if there are any present now, or whether there have been any problems in this area in the past.

Common pathologies would be:

Cold sores - painful sores around the mouth, usually found on the lips. These are caused by a virus.

Gingivitis - where the gums become red and inflamed. This is a very common form of gum disease.

Halitosis - commonly known as bad breath. This causes the breath to smell unpleasant. It is caused by bacteria in the mouth.

A mouth ulcer - an open sore on the lining of the mouth.

Oral thrush - a yeast infection of the mouth that causes white patches in the mouth.

Toothache - pain or discomfort in one or more teeth; it can also occur in the gums. It is typified by radiating pain from the affected tooth or gum that can also affect the face, neck or ears.

Remember to state that reflexology is a sensitive therapy that can pick up current issues and past issues – it does not mean there are any major problems and may relate to a physical or an emotional imbalance in the body.

If the mouth reflex area - also covering jaw, teeth and throat - is out of balance, consider:

Physical prompts:

- Do they have any current pain in their mouth, jaw, throat or teeth?

- Are they prone to any conditions or infections in their mouth, jaw, throat or teeth?

- Do they hold tension in their jaw when they are stressed?

- Do they suffer with a dry mouth – perhaps when they are stressed?

- Are they aware if they grind their teeth at night?

The skin

Location in body

The skin is the body's largest organ and can be found covering all external surfaces of the body except the eyes.

How to treat:
As the skin is on top of all parts of the body to some degree, it receives stimulation and treatment throughout the standard reflexology session.

Physiological action:

The skin has three layers; the epidermis, the dermis and the subcutaneous layer.

Together, these layers fulfil the following functions:

- Secretion of sebum (an oily substance), which combines with perspiration on the surface of the skin to form a natural skin moisturiser, whilst also protecting against bacteria.
- Heat regulation, through:
  - » vasodilation (capillaries near the skin's surface widening to allow more blood through them so the heat can be lost to the surrounding air).
  - » perspiration (the release and evaporation of sweat from the skin's surface).
  - » hairs erecting (to keep a layer of warm air trapped near the surface of the skin).
  - » hairs flattening (to avoid the layer of warm air being trapped).
  - » vasoconstriction (capillaries near the skin's surface becoming narrower to restrict heat loss to the surrounding air).
- Absorption of some oils and drugs.
- Protection of the internal organs by keeping micro-organisms out and forming a barrier against the sun's rays.
- Elimination of waste products of the body through sweat.
- Sensation of heat, cold, pain, pressure and touch through nerve endings in the dermis.
- Vitamin D production.
- Melanin production to aid protection from the sun's rays.

Physical problems or illnesses to be aware of:

When thinking of the skin, it is important to think of all the issues that might affect the skin and check to see if there are any present now, or whether there have been any problems with the skin in the past.

Common pathologies would be:

Acne - a chronic skin disease that affects many adolescents to some extent, causing small spots or lumps to be present on the skin (most commonly on the face, back or chest).

Alopecia - sudden, often temporary, hair loss.

Athlete's foot - a fungal condition that occurs between the toes, which makes the skin inflamed, moist, flaky, itchy and/or painful.

Boils - red, painful lumps on the skin at the site of an infected hair follicle. A collection of them together is called a carbuncle.

Cellulitis - an infection of the deeper layers of the skin, causing it to become hot, painful, red and swollen.

Chilblains - small, itchy, painful, red-purple swellings on the fingers, caused by some of the blood flow leaking through the walls of a blood vessel as it dilates after it has narrowed due to the cold. They can also be present on the toes, nose or other extremities.

Corns and calluses - hard, thickened areas of skin on the feet, most commonly caused by prolonged periods of pressure or friction on a small area of skin.

176

Contact dermatitis/ eczema - a condition that causes inflammation of the skin. With contact dermatitis, this is normally caused by allergies, irritants or exposure to a substance that causes an abnormal reaction from the immune system.

Dandruff - a common condition that affects the skin of the scalp, which causes small (but visible) flakes of skin to shed.

Folliculitis - most commonly caused by bacteria infecting pre-existing damage to the hair follicle (e.g. friction, shaving, insect bites or a blocked follicle) and is characterised by itchy or painful redness, with small red pimples in the upper part of the follicles which may crust over. This is called

Barber's Itch when found on the beard area of the face. Folliculitis can be found in any hairy area of the body, not just the face or scalp.

Heel fissures - cracked, split heels which are commonly caused by dry skin.

Hives - raised, red, itchy patches on the skin, which most commonly result from an allergic reaction.

Hyperhidrosis - normally excessive sweating in specific areas, although it can affect the whole body in rarer cases. It most commonly affects the feet, armpits, hands or face.

Impetigo - a common bacterial skin condition where small blisters appear, which then burst, leaving moist yellow patches behind, which then dry to a crust. It is most common in babies and small children, although it can affect anyone. Impetigo is very contagious.

Keratosis pilaris - where the skin is rough and bumpy all the time, looking like chicken skin. It is harmless.

Melanoma - a form of skin cancer, most commonly caused by over-exposure to UV rays.

Pediculosis - where lice are living on the skin's surface, often causing itchy bites.

Psoriasis - an autoimmune condition that most commonly causes silvery or red scaly rashes to be present on the skin's surface.

Ringworm - a fungal infection of the skin, where the fungal growths follow a ring-like pattern, causing a round red or silvery rash with a patch of normal coloured skin in the middle.

Scabies - where little mites burrow into the skin, most commonly in the webbing between fingers and toes. Their excrement causes itching, and their burrowing action causes tiny silvery or brown lines to appear on the skin's surface.

Scars - patches or lines of tissue which remain in the location of a wound after it has healed, where the body has produced more collagen than is needed to make the new skin to knit together the wound.

Sebaceous cysts - harmless swelling under the skin commonly caused by the inflammation or blockage of a hair follicle, causing a build-up of dead skin and sebum under the skin's surface.

Shingles - a painful rash along the path of a nerve, caused by the chickenpox virus. It is also known as herpes zoster.

Vitiligo - where white patches appear on the skin, caused by a lack of melanocyte cells.

Warts and verrucae - small, horny non-cancerous growths on the skin, caused by a virus. These are contagious.

Remember to state that reflexology is a sensitive therapy that can pick up current issues and past issues – it does not mean there are any major problems and may relate to a physical or an emotional imbalance in the body.

The skin reflexes are present throughout the feet; however, you could consider:

Physical prompts:

- Do they have or have they ever had any skin problems?

- Do they have sensitive skin?

Emotional links: Sensory system

If physical issues are present, the emotional involvement may still be important as part of the illness. If none of these are present, then it is even more important to consider emotional blocks.

Key area: about connection to and communicating with their senses – feelings, inner sense (sixth sense/ intuition/ knowing).

Be aware as you listen, not to tell them how you think they should move forward, but instead ask useful questions to allow them to explore the ideas.

Exploring possible emotional reasons for reflexes that are out of balance has to be handled with great sensitivity, and it can be presented purely as one school of thought. It may be that it is not suitable to share this information with your client, but it might help you understand why the reflex is imbalanced. You will need to use careful judgement as to whether to share this information.

The eyes: *how the person sees their life from their inner point of view.*

- Is there something going on in their life that perhaps they don't want to see?

- Do they need to 'open their eyes' to something?

- What is it that they are not seeing in their current situation?

The ears: *what is being heard and how that affects the person.*

- Is something being said that they don't like or do not want to hear?

- Are they listening to and trusting their intuition?

The nose: *what is being faced head on (as the nose is centre face) and the way that is being interpreted.*

- Are they getting a 'whiff' of things not being right? Or smelling out a different story?

- What's got up their nose recently?

The mouth: *this is about what we take in and reject in communication terms.*

- Are they speaking up and putting their view forward?

- Are they swallowing any situation because they believe they can't change it? Is there something they could do to change it?

- Are they able to express easily their core beliefs and ideas?

- Are they speaking their truths and values or someone else's?

The skin: *this represents your reaction to life*

- Are issues getting under their skin?

- Are they irritated by something?

Appendix 1: A quick reference guide to all the body systems

The Cardiovascular system

Physiological= transports life-giving components around the body.
Emotional= all about love and being loved.

Heart

Physical prompts:

- Do they get cold feet and hands?
- Are they aware of any circulatory problems now or in the past?
- Have they had any physical problems with their heart?
- Do they have any areas of venous stagnation – blue or painful areas in the legs for example?
- Do they suffer from Raynaud's Syndrome – white or blue painful fingers when cold?

Emotional prompts:

- What fills the client with love?
- What does the client love?
- Is the amount that they love equal to the amount that they are loved? Is one easier than the other for them?
- Is it safe to love and be loved? *Many have been deeply hurt and as a result fear loving and being loved due to past experiences including rejection and deep hurt.*
- Do they feel that they have enough love?

The lymphatic system

Physiological= major role in the immune defence of the body.

Emotional= the ability to get rid of what no longer serves us.

Physical prompts:

- Have they had any major infections in their life?

- Have they had any recent infections such as a cold or flu?

- Do they have any signs of 'killing off' infections such as a sore throat or sore glands?

- Do they have any swollen parts of their body?

- Have they had any major operations?

- Have they been in contact with anyone who has a bad infection? *Their body could be in protection mode.*

Emotional prompts:

The lymphatic system is all about every kind of 'letting go' physically, emotionally, energetically or spiritually. Any fluid (lymph) that builds up represents withheld emotion (water equals emotion; e/motion equals energy in motion). Consider:

- What are they holding on to? (As opposed to having processed and let go of).

- Do they need to let go of something?

- Do they feel a bit stagnant?

As lymph is only moved due to the movement of skeletal muscles, if there is no movement, the lymph (chi/energy) stagnates.

The area of the lymphatic fluid build-up will give more information of what the theme of their issue may be about. For example, swollen ankles equal withheld emotion and lack of flow to do with what a person stands for and how they stride out or forward.

The endocrine system

Physiological = the process of secreting hormones into the blood circulation.

Emotional = in general, this relates to messages being sent and received.

The hypothalamus

Physical prompts:

If the hypothalamus reflex is out of balance, remember that its primary function is to maintain homeostasis and as such, it is involved in many necessary processes of the body including behavioural, autonomic and endocrine functions, such as metabolism, growth and development.

Consider if there are issues with:

- Physiological functions such as temperature regulation (may include hot flushes), thirst, hunger, sleep, fluid balance, blood pressure, mood, sex drive.

- Endocrine functions such as metabolism and growth and development in children.

- Physical and psychological effects of oxytocin – frequently referred to as the 'love hormone', oxytocin has an effect on bonding, stress, anxiety and depression, social skills, breastfeeding and childbirth etc.

Emotional prompts:

The pituitary and hypothalamus are all about our sixth sense. They are the houses of intuition or inner knowing. They are our internal radar and keep us connected to our intuition. When the pituitary and hypothalamus are working well and in balance, we find it easier to be connected to all of our senses and our intuition.

- How is the client's intuition functioning at the moment? Are they trying to avoid it?

The pituitary gland

Physical prompts:

- Have they been generally feeling 'out of sorts' hormone-wise?

- Are they very stressed?

N.B. High levels of stress can produce a negative feedback loop on the pituitary gland causing it to function less efficiently. The pituitary is also a very busy and important gland, so it is often slightly out of balance for no discernible reason.

Emotional prompts:

The pituitary and hypothalamus are all about our sixth sense. They are the houses of intuition or inner knowing. They are our internal radar and keep us connected to our intuition. When the pituitary and hypothalamus are working well and in balance, we find it easier to be connected to all of our senses and our intuition.

- How is the client's intuition functioning at the moment? Are they trying to avoid it?

The adrenal glands

Physical prompts:

- Is the client very stressed at the moment or have they had periods of high stress in the past?

- Are they waking frequently in the night or finding it difficult to wake up in the morning?

- Do they feel their heart racing for no apparent reason?

N.B. rule out overuse of stimulants such as caffeine with the last point.

Emotional prompts:

This is about coping with life and life shocks, fears and anxiety. The adrenals are also associated with speed, a speedy life and being able to respond immediately. It is to do with pace of life. If the adrenals are over working, the person may be living a life that is moving too fast.

The adrenal gland/ kidney reflexes are also located on the horizontal zone connected to 'doing' energy and working life issues.

- Is the client very competitive? Even perhaps against themselves?

- How are things at work for them?

- What is it that they are doing or that is being done that is causing them stress?

- Are they doing too many things rather than focusing on just one?

- Can they swap activity to inactivity – busy head (thoughts) to calm thoughts, highly charged to very chilled?

The pineal gland

Physical prompts:

- Are they having trouble getting to sleep or staying asleep?

- Are they a frequent long-haul flyer?

- Do they have or have they had in the past any periods of jet lag?

- Do they do shift work?

N.B. you could mention the importance of getting light into the eyes for resetting the 'body clock'. Going out in the light every day is important , as is taking off glasses if they are worn, as they can block some of the critical wavelengths of light.

Emotional prompts:

The pineal atrophies over time and relates to keeping connection with the bigger picture. It is our connection to our "meaning of life."

- Are they feeling disconnected from the world at the moment?

The thyroid

Physical prompts:

- Do they often feel cold, have a lack of energy and put weight on easily?

- Do they feel hot, full of energy and lose weight at the drop of a hat?

N.B. these can be indications of hypo- or hyper- thyroid issues. If the client is experiencing these symptoms, you should advise your client to explain their symptoms to their GP and then tests may be offered.

Emotional prompts:

The thyroid is the centre of our communication. It's our verbal and non-verbal, internal and external communication. It is the words (and tone) that we use to speak out into the world and the words (and tone) that we use to speak in our own heads; the actual words plus body language, expressions and ways of living. Thyroid energy is all about communication in every possible way. Taking the communication link further, the thyroid reflex also indicates the emotional area to reflect self-esteem issues:

- How is their self-esteem at the moment?

- What one thing specifically could they do today to boost their self-esteem?

If the thyroid is overactive, it's an indication that there is too much going on. If it is underactive then stagnation may be the cause. Not knowing and not being able to communicate themselves as they are, can cause stagnation and underactivity.

- Are they having problems communicating with someone in particular?

The parathyroid

Physical prompts:

- Is the client prone to episodes of cramp?

- Has the client been diagnosed with osteoporosis?

- Is the client a menopausal woman, who is at higher risk?

Emotional prompts:

This is related to feeling strong.

- Are they feeling that their strength is being sapped by something?

- Do they need to conserve their strength?

The thymus

Physical prompts:

- Do they find it easy to get rid of any colds or infections?

- Do they have any indications that their immune system may be low?

Emotional prompts:

This is the centre of our loving connection to self and our body. The centre of the immune system is directly connected to our love of self and others.

- Are they finding it hard to love themselves at the moment?

The pancreas

Physical prompts:

If the pancreas reflex is out of balance, remember this could relate to endocrine or exocrine function; consider:

- Do they get any right sided abdominal pain?
- Do they get regular nausea, vomiting or had any weight loss?
- Are they aware if they have any problems with blood sugar levels?
- Has their diet changed, especially changes to the amount of sugar they eat?
- Do they ever feel like they could faint when they haven't eaten?
- Do they go to the loo more than usual?

* N.B. these could be symptoms of diabetes, so advise your client to take these symptoms to their GP where they might be offered further tests.

Emotional prompts:

The pancreas *represents the processing of life and relates to how sweet it is – or not. Enzymes that the pancreas produces aid digestion and so this relates to the ability of the person to be able to break life down into small parcels/particles.*

Sometimes life is not sweet or the sweetness is lost. Looking at the small parts of life can make it easier to find the sweet things (nice things or small aspects of life that are okay). An imbalance in the pancreas which leads to more challenges with blood sugar levels can be caused by someone receiving a shock of significant proportion.

Shock can impact the function of the pancreas and the physical knock-on effects can be picked up within two years of the shock occurring.

The pancreas relates to confidence and creativity. Shock can negatively impact these. The resolution is to take tiny steps forward to increase

creativity and confidence. With an increase of both of these, the person will have more energy, strength and ability to cope with any further life shocks. Being able to cope keeps the sweetness of life. Creatively keeping and re-finding or reconnecting with sweet moments is very empowering to anything pancreatic.

- In terms of what they are doing or what is being done, how can the client bring the sweetness back to what they are doing?

- How are they feeling about what they are doing or what is being done?

The ovaries and testes

Physical prompts:

For the ovaries:

- Do they have any problems that could be related to their periods?

For the testes:

- Do they have any problems that could be related to their prostate?

- Do they have any problems urinating?

- Have they noticed any functional problems?

Emotional prompts:

These reflexes are both related to reproducing self. Do you want to replicate you? Is your life something you would like to replicate? It's about passing something forward for humanity to benefit by. If someone is unhappy with who they are and does not wish to replicate that or pass it forward, they are more likely to experience endocrine issues relating to the reproductive areas, and this can be eased when someone finds more peace, love and acceptance for themselves and 'who vs. how' they are.

Issues around the endocrine system may also be about creativity:

- Are they accessing their creative side enough?

- If they could create anything, what would they like to create?

- Are they unhappy about who they are?

The uterus area is representative of expansion and space, so you could consider:

- Are they planning a period of expansion?

- Do they have enough space to grow? (their family for example?)

- If fertility related, do they have enough room in their life for a(nother) baby?

The excretory system

Physiological= the process of filtering the body of its waste and the disposal of that waste.

Emotional= represents support impacting on family or private life.

The kidney

Physical prompts:

- Do they have or have they had any problems with their kidneys?

- Do they have or have they had any pain in their back around the level of their waist?

- Do they have or have they had any problems urinating?

- How has their water intake been recently?

- Have they noticed if their urine has changed in colour recently e.g. darker than normal?

- Have they been sweating more than usual? Has it been hot, have they been doing a lot of exercise or having hot sweats? All of these can mean that water is being lost through the skin, concentrating the waste products.

Emotional prompts:

The kidney represents 'going with the flow' of life. It also represents the house of fear because if you are frightened then it is difficult to 'go with the flow'. Its about learning to go with YOUR flow.

- Are they fearful of something in their life?

- Are they fighting against going with the flow?

- Do they sometimes feel that they are 'swimming upstream' against issues?

An alternative view of this is that it represents 'the way you are thinking about how you are feeling is impacting on what you are doing or what is being done'.

- How are they feeling about what they are doing?

- The kidney can also represent crying inside or unshed tears.

- Do they need to have a good cry about something?

The ureter

Physical prompts:

- Do they or have they had any problems urinating/passing water?

- How has their water intake been recently?

- Have they noticed if their urine has changed in colour recently e.g. darker than normal, as this may irritate the ureter tubes?

Emotional prompts:

This is related to the ability to let let go (or not!)

- Are they having issues with the letting go of some thought or emotion?

- Is there something in their life that they need to let go of?

The bladder

Physical prompts:

- Do they have or have they had any problems with their bladder such as infections?

- Have they noticed if they are urinating/ passing water more often?

  If Yes: Does it hurt, feel like it's burning or feel itchy when they urinate or do they feel like they don't empty their bladder fully? If these symptom persist for more than a few days then the client should arrange to see their GP to discuss their symptoms, as it may be a sign of an infection.

- Have they noticed if their urine has changed in colour recently e.g. darker than normal?

- How is their water intake?

- Have they been sweating more than usual - has it been hot, have they been doing a lot of exercise or having hot sweats? All of these can mean that water is being lost through the skin, concentrating the waste products.

Emotional prompts:

This relates to everything about being truly fed up – in other words – 'peed off'. When someone has an issue with their bladder, it is very often at a time when something has made them feel this way.

- Have they been feeling fed up or peed off with someone or something recently?

It's also about holding onto things and being unable to let go or letting go in an extreme fashion. Bladder incontinence is when the general pressure of life is causing someone to be peed off (fed up) and something (the bladder) gives under pressure.

Bladder retention problems are when someone is trying to hang onto their flow of life, when life does not feel free-flowing. Urine is about flow – too fast, lack of, or painful.

- Are they feeling as though their life has stagnated?

- Is their life moving too fast?

- Have they been sweating more than usual - has it been hot, have they been doing a lot of exercise or having hot sweats? All of these can mean that water is being lost through the skin, concentrating the waste products.

The urethra

Physical prompts:

- Does it hurt them, feel like it burns or feel itchy when they urinate?

191

- Is there a discharge from the urethra?

- Do they have any pain in their lower pelvic region?

- Do they find they have difficulty urinating?

If these symptoms persist then the client should arrange to see their GP to discuss their symptoms, as it may be a sign of an infection or blockage.

Emotional prompts:

This spans over two emotional areas: those of family and work.

a) The way they are thinking about how they are feeling impacting on what they are doing or what is being done.

b) The way they are thinking about their self-esteem or core beliefs and ideas is impacting on their private life.

- How are they feeling about what is being done?

- What's happening at work?

- Is their self-esteem impacting on how they relate to others?

- How are things between them and their family or partner?

The digestive system

Physiological= the processes involved in the breaking down of food and absorption of nutrients and with the elimination of waste products.

Emotional= the digestion and enjoyment of life.

The mouth

Physical prompts:

- Do they have any current pain in their mouth, jaw, throat or teeth?
- Are they prone to any conditions or infections in their mouth, jaw, throat or teeth?
- Do they hold tension in their jaw when they are stressed?
- Do they suffer with a dry mouth – perhaps when they are stressed?
- Are they aware if they grind their teeth at night?
- If the jaw is out of balance, see if the client has had a hip problem. The two can be linked.

Emotional prompts:

This is about what we take in and reject in communication terms.

- Are they speaking up, putting their view forward?
- Are they swallowing any situation because they believe they can't change it?
- Is there something they could do to change it?
- Are they able to express easily their core beliefs and ideas?
- Are they speaking their truths and values or someone else's?

The stomach

Physical prompts:

- Are they aware of any issues with their stomach?
- Have they had any nausea or vomiting recently?
- Do they ever get a sour, unpleasant taste in their mouth?

- Do they get 'butterflies' in their tummy when they are stressed?

- Have they changed their diet recently?

N.B. Also consider if there is anything in their lifestyle which may be causing inflammation or irritation in the stomach lining (but as yet is asymptomatic) such as excessive alcohol consumption, regular use of Aspirin, Ibuprofen or other non-steroidal anti-inflammatory drugs (NSAIDs). This will have to be handled sensitively (especially if there is excessive alcohol consumption); judge how well you know your client and then consider a phrase such as:

- "It may be that the painkillers you are on are causing a little irritation – do you always take these after you have eaten?"

- "You mentioned your alcohol consumption is quite high and alcohol can irritate the stomach lining, which is possibly what I am picking up."

Emotional prompts:

This is about how we stomach or cope with life and start to absorb and "chew life over" – a process started with chewing in the mouth.

- Is there something that they are finding difficult to stomach?

- Was there a situation in their past that was difficult to stomach?

The liver

Physical prompts:

194

- Are they aware of any issues with their liver?

- Has there been a change in the amount of alcohol they have drunk recently?

- Have they had any infections recently, especially of the digestive system?

- Have they made any changes to their diet, especially of fatty foods?

- Have they increased their physical activity? *This may mean the liver is having to release more energy.*

- Are they on medications which may be broken down by the liver?

Emotional prompts:

This is about keeping in anger about something.

- Have there have been any situations recently where they have felt angry?

- Have they ever felt that they had to suppress their anger?

The gall bladder

Physical prompts:

- Are they aware of any issues with their gall bladder?

- Has there been a change in their diet, especially an increase in fatty foods?

- Do they feel uncomfortable after eating fatty foods?

Emotional prompts:

This is about making decisions.

- Are they having trouble making a decision about something?

- Do they have too many decisions to make?

The pancreas

Physical prompts:

- Do they get any right sided abdominal pain?

- Do they get regular nausea, vomiting or had any weight loss?

- Are they aware if they have any problems with blood sugar levels?

- Has their diet changed, especially changes to the amount of sugar they eat?

- Do they ever feel like they could faint when they haven't eaten?

- Do they go to the loo more than usual?

N.B. these could be symptoms of a medical problem, so advise your client to take these symptoms to their GP where they might be offered further tests.

Emotional prompts:

This is all about the sweetness of life (or not). It's about digesting life and creating the sweet balance of life.

- Have they felt the sweetness disappearing from their life recently?

- Was there a situation in the past when they felt that sweetness was drained from their life?

The general intestinal area

Emotional prompts:

- How are things at home for the client?

- Are there issues to do with their family or private life?

- Are they walking the easiest path that perhaps doesn't exactly fit them?

The small intestine

Physical prompts:

- Have they had any problems with their bowels recently?

- Are they prone to constipation or diarrhoea?

- Have they changed their diet recently?

- When they are stressed does it affect their bowels?

- Do they ever feel bloated?

- Do they sit for long periods with a poor posture, which may be affecting the nerve supply to the intestines?

N.B. Also consider if there is anything in their lifestyle which may be causing inflammation or irritation in the small intestine but as yet is asymptomatic, such as poor diet (lack of fibre, fatty or fried foods, processed foods etc). This may be a time to address their diet, especially if they are feeling tired or stressed.

Emotional prompts:

This is related to the absorption of life, and also sits in the area of family and home, so there may be cross references to home issues.

- Are they finding something difficult to absorb?

- Are they hanging on to something that they should let go of?

The appendix

Physical prompts:

- Do they get any dull aches or sharp pains on the right side of their abdomen?

- Do they sit for long periods with a poor posture, which may be affecting the nerve supply to the abdominal area?

N.B. It is essential to reassure clients that an imbalance here does not mean that they have appendicitis, but may just indicate a minor irritation in or around the appendix or ileocaecal valve.

If the pain remains constant or becomes more acute they should be referred to a GP. Tell your client to make an appointment with their GP to discuss their symptoms. Reassure them that this is probably something minor but is worth checking out.

Emotional prompts:

This is all about the ability to move forwards and not backwards.

- Are they having trouble moving forwards with something?

- Are they a bit stuck?

The large intestine

Physical prompts:

- Have they had any problems with their bowels recently?

- Are they prone to constipation or diarrhoea?

- Have they changed their diet recently? *Even if they have improved their diet it can take time for the digestive system to become used to this.*

- When they are stressed does it tend to affect their bowels?

- Do they ever feel bloated?

- Do they sit for long periods with a poor posture, which may be affecting the nerve supply to the intestines?

Emotional prompts:

The ascending colon is about taking up life, of beginning to process life, to be able to process and filter /digest and then be creatively themselves.

- Is there anything they are having problems with in their life?

- Are they feeling stagnated creatively?

- Can they be the person they feel they really are?

- Have they had problems in the past in moving forward and taking the next steps?

The transverse colon is about honouring the self, of being creative, of being courageous and able to cope with life shocks (or not!)

- Do they need to be brave about something to feel really themselves?

The descending colon is about staying grounded and able to physically process and let go of what is not helpful to each unique individual and the person that only they can be in the world.

- Do they have emotions that need to be released or let go? *If so, then to let go will be healing. Note: they may need to visit a counsellor/ their GP for help in doing this.*

The rectum/anus

Physical prompts:

- Are they prone to constipation?

- Do they have any pain when they open their bowels?

- Do they have, or have they ever suffered with piles/haemorrhoids?

- (If a the client is a woman with children) did you have any issues with piles during pregnancy?

Emotional prompts

This is related to our sense of security and plans for the future.

- Are they feeling insecure about their plans for the future?

The musculoskeletal system

Physiological= provides structures to the body that allow it to connect, move and respond.

Emotional= support, moving forward.

The head

Physical prompts:

- Have they had a headache recently or is this something that they tend to suffer with?

- Do they carry tension in their neck, as this can also cause tension in the head area?

- Have they been under a lot of stress recently?

- Do they have a busy brain?

- Have they had a cold recently? *(especially if sinus reflexes come up)*

- Have they been on a long haul flight? *Aircraft pressure can change how these function (especially if the sinus/ eustacian tube reflexes come up).*

- Have they had any dizziness recently or issues with their ears? *(especially if the eustacian tubes and ear reflexes are out of balance).*

Emotional prompts:

The head represents the brain area, so ask questions about thinking:

- What are they spending lots of time thinking about?

- What do they believe?

- Is there something affecting their core beliefs and ideas?

The neck

Physical prompts:

- Do they have any stiffness or pain in their neck?

- If they are stressed, do they carry their tension in their neck and shoulders?

- Do they sit at a computer for long periods – is their working position correct? *If they hunch over or look down at a keyboard, this can put strain on the neck muscles.*

- An imbalance in the neck reflex is common in times of high stress – might this be the reason?

- How would they describe their posture when they are sitting, standing and walking – is their head held upright with their shoulders back?

- Do they do any activities that involve them moving their neck repeatedly such as swimming? *Whilst swimming is very good exercise, if they swim with their head held out of the water, this places strain on the neck.*

- How do they answer their phone? *People often tilt their head to one side when answering a phone, which puts stress on the neck muscles when done regularly.*

- Do they carry a heavy bag on one shoulder?

Emotional prompts:

The neck represents the connection between head (thoughts) and heart (feelings). People with neck problems often have a disconnect between the two.

- Do they feel their head and heart are flowing in the same direction?

- What are they not saying that needs to be said?

Alternatively, it can represent an expression:

- Who is being a pain in the neck?

Hard skin on the neck reflex may indicate not wanting to talk about a situation, so it may be sensitive. Consider:

- Do they have something on their mind that they aren't able to express?

The shoulder

Physical prompts:

- Do they have or have they had any problems with their shoulders?

- Do they get any stiffness or pain in their shoulders?

- If they are stressed, do they carry their tension in their neck and shoulders?

- Do they sit at a computer for long periods – is their working position correct? *If they hunch over a keyboard, shoulders can become tense; it is important they regularly lift their head and pull their shoulders back.*

- Tense shoulders are common in times of high stress – could this be the reason for the imbalance?

- How would they describe their posture when they are sitting, standing and walking – is their head held upright with their shoulders back?

- Do they tend to carry a heavy bag on one shoulder?

Emotional prompts:

This represents shouldering responsibilities, so consider:

- How much responsibility is resting on their shoulders right now?

- Can they think of one way, specifically, that they could make their responsibilities easier to deal with?

- What is it they feel or are told they "should" be doing but don't really want to?

The elbows

Physical prompts:

- Do they have or have they had any problems with their elbow?

- Do they or have they had any issues with their arm?

- Do they spend long periods of time on repetitive moves that involve bending the elbow, e.g. tennis or golf?

Emotional prompts:

The elbow is related to flexibility and direction:

- Do they need to change direction?

- Are they feeling inflexible emotionally?

- How can they find ways to more easily go with the flow?

The sacroiliac joint

Physical prompts:

- Have they had any lower back or hip problems now or in the past?

- Have they had any slight slips or trips recently?

- Have they been pregnant?

The pelvis

Physical prompts:

- Do they have, or have they had, any problems with their pelvic area?

- Do they think this is an area where they hold tension? *A lot of people stand with their glutes tight and tense.*

- Do they have any problems with their digestion (bowels)?

- Do they have any problems with their periods? *Sometimes with heavy periods or issues with the uterus, the pelvic area may be tense.*

- Do they or have they had any issues with their lower back? *This may relate to tension in the pelvic girdle*

- Have they been doing exercise that might have affected their pelvis?

- If they had a pregnancy - did they have any back problems or pubic symphysis disorder?

Emotional prompts:

This represents grounding and sense of security in moving forward:
- How secure do they feel about their plans for the future?

- What are they planning?

If there is hard skin here, you can be sure the person is feeling insecure about their plans for the future, so instead consider:

- Is there one thing specifically that they can put in place to allow themselves to feel more secure about putting their plans into action?

The leg

Physical prompts:

- Do they have or have they had any problems with their legs?

- Is there an excess or lack of exercise? *This may be why they are feeling tension here.*

- Do they have or have they had any problems with their hips or knees? *This will affect the flow of energy in this zone – sometimes it can even be blocked energy from higher in the zone e.g. shoulder.*

Emotional prompts:

This is about how they stand, progress and move in life.

- Are they having problems with where or how they stand in life?

The knees

Physical prompts:

- Do they have or have they had any problems with their knees?

- Do they do any regular activity which requires bending repeatedly?

- Is there an excess or lack of exercise? *This may be why they are feeling tension here.*

- Do they have or have they had any problems with their hips or legs? *This will affect the flow of energy in this zone – sometimes it can even be blocked energy from higher in the zone e.g. shoulder.*

Emotional prompts:

The knee is all about moving forward.

- Do they have plans that they can't quite put in motion?

- What can they do to allow themselves to put their plans into action?

The respiratory system

Physical = the ability to receive or inhale (oxygen) and release or exhale (carbon dioxide).

Emotional = represents the ability to receive and release in the emotional parts of life.

Physical prompts:

- Do they currently have any problems with their lungs or chest?

- Have they had any major problems in the past?

- Are they prone to any lung or breathing problems such as chest infections, asthma etc?

- Do they get any aerobic exercise which allows the lungs to work efficiently? *Be aware, this could be a sign of excessive exercise or too little.*

- Do they hunch over a computer, which may restrict the flow of blood and energy through the lungs?

- Do they have allergies and if so, have they been in contact with that allergen recently?

- Do they smoke?

Emotional prompts:

204

- Do they feel as though they are holding on to any emotions?
- How are they feeling?
- What emotion are they keeping in?
- What emotion might they be keeping to themselves that they don't want others to know?
- To whom do they feel they can't show how they are feeling?
- How long have they been hiding their feelings?
- How do they enjoy and flow with life?
- How much enjoyment do they have in their life?
- Have they been through any major process of grieving in their life? Do they feel they have released all the emotions attached to this time?

The reproductive system

Physiological= The production of a new human being.

Emotional= Grounding and the emotions around the replication of self. This can also include how secure you are feeling.

The fallopian tubes

Physical prompts:

- Do they have very painful periods? *If yes, have they ever seen their GP about these?*

- Do they sit for long periods with a poor posture, which may be affecting the nerve supply to the pelvic area?

- Have they had any problems with their reproductive system in the past?

N.B. If they are seeing you regarding conception, you can ask if they have had any tests e.g. ultra sound scan, laparoscopy etc.

The uterus

Physical prompts:

- How are their periods? Would they describe them as particularly heavy or painful?

- Do they get any pain or bloating in their abdomen? *If yes, have they ever seen their GP about this?*

- Do they currently have their period?

- Do they sit for long periods with a poor posture, which may be affecting the nerve supply to the pelvic area?

N.B. If they are seeing you regarding conception, you can ask if they have had any tests e.g. ultra sound scan, laparoscopy etc.

The cervix

Physical prompts:

- Have they been aware of any problems with their cervix before? *This could be during pregnancy or not.*

Be aware that the cervix is connected to the vagina, and sometimes if thrush, vaginal dryness etc. has been an issue, the cervix may show up as well.

The vagina

Physical prompts:

- Do they feel they have any problems in this area? *They may have had thrush, or may have some vaginal dryness – this is more common in the menopause.*

Note: these are not reflexes that all therapists include in their treatments. If you do include these you will need to feel confident to handle these conversations as they are of a personal nature. You may wish to wait until the client has had a couple of treatments and is more comfortable with you.

The epididymis

Physical prompts:

- Do they have, or have they ever had any discomfort in the pelvic region?

- Do they sit for long periods with a poor posture, which may be affecting the nerve supply to the pelvis?

N.B. If they are seeing you regarding conception, you can ask if they have had any tests e.g. semen analysis, and ask what the results were.

The Vas deferens

Physical prompts:

- Do they have, or have they ever had any discomfort in the pelvic region?

- Do they sit for long periods with a poor posture, which may be affecting the nerve supply to the pelvis?

N.B. If they are seeing you regarding conception, you can ask if they have had any tests e.g. semen analysis, and ask what the results were.

The prostate

Physical prompts:

- Do they have any problems urinating? **

- Do they feel the need to go to the toilet frequently? **

- Do they have, or have they ever had any discomfort in the pelvic region?

- Do they sit for long periods with a poor posture, which may be affecting the nerve supply to the pelvis?

*** If the answer to this is yes, they should be referred to a GP. Tell your client to make an appointment to discuss his symptoms. Reassure him that this is probably something minor but is worth checking out.*

Emotional prompts: the reproductive system as a whole

These are about grounding and links to base chakra, as well as replication of self. This can also include how secure you are feeling.

- If they could truly be themselves, here on Earth, who would they be? How would they be living, experiencing life?

- What changes do they need to make or could they make to be more of who they really are?

- How secure or insecure are they feeling about the future?

- What one thing specifically could they do to help themselves to feel more secure and allow them to move forward to take the next steps?

The nervous system

Physiological= co-ordination and integration of information which then influences activities.

Emotional= a central link to our core beliefs, ideas and self-esteem.

Physical prompts:

- Do they consider themselves to be an anxious person?

- Are they under high levels of stress?

- Do they think they have a high tolerance for stress?

- Do they need to exercise and feel unwell if they don't? *This can indicate a high fight or flight response stimulation, because the arms and legs are full of pumping blood which has to be released by exercise and therefore may be an indicator of high stress levels.*

- Do they suffer from headaches of any sort?

- Do they have, or have they had in the past, any diagnosed illnesses relating to their nervous system?

Emotional prompts:

The brain represents core beliefs, ideas, and also self-esteem. If someone is constantly knocking your beliefs, your self-esteem will suffer. If you find your client fixates about one specific belief, you can open their eyes by considering wider issues, such as:

208

- Is there something or someone that is getting on their nerves at the moment?

- Have they had a traumatic or emotional episode in the past? If so, do they think that how they feel now might be related to that time?

- Do they need to let go of past trauma? *This may require extra help from other health professionals*

- Saying "That's one solution; can you think of any other solutions?"

Reflexologists can help people with CNS issues by helping them to focus on the 'now', feel confident in themselves and to notice and be grateful for what is right (rather than what might be wrong).

The spine/ spinal cord

Physical prompts:

- Are they very anxious or stressed?
- Do they suffer from the sensation of pins and needles anywhere in the body?
- Do they have any feelings of numbness anywhere in the body?

Emotional prompts:

The spine is our core and central support – it relates to support received, but also to how we stand up to things, people and situations.

- Are they getting enough support?
- Where would they like more support in their life right now?
- Who might they need to stand up to in their life?

Lower spine issues relate to the biggest core worry that is often at the root of things for most people in the western world, and can represent a lack of financial support.

- Do they feel unsupported, specifically in the financial area of their life?

The sensory system

Physiological= awareness of the world around you through the senses.

Emotional= about connection to and communicating feelings, inner sense (sixth sense/ intuition/ knowing).

The eyes

Physical prompts:

- Do they have or have they had any problems with their eyes?

- Do they work for long periods on a computer or other types of screens?

- Do they wear glasses and if so, have they had an eye test recently?

- Do they have any sinus problems at the moment?

- Do they suffer from hay fever or itchy eyes?

Emotional prompts:

These represent how the person sees their life from their inner point of view.

- Is there something going on in their life that perhaps they don't want to see?

- Do they need to 'open their eyes' to something?

- What is it that they are not seeing in their current situation?

The ears

Physical prompts:

- Do they have or have they had any problems with their ears?

- Do they ever get a feeling of dizziness?

- Do their ears feel as if they are blocked?

- Do they work around loud noises or listen to loud music?

Emotional prompts:

These represent what is being heard and how that affects the person.

- Is something being said that they don't like or do not want to hear?

- Are they listening to and trusting their intuition?

The nose

Physical prompts:

- Do they have or have they had any problems with their nose, such as itchiness, sneezing, feeling of a blocked nose, or nose bleeds?

- Are they prone to getting blocked sinuses?

- Do they suffer from allergies or hay fever?

Emotional prompts:

This represents what is being faced head on (as the nose is centre face) and the way in which it is being interpreted.

- Are they getting a 'whiff' of things not being right? Or smelling out a different story?

- What's got up their nose recently?

The mouth

Physical prompts:

If the mouth reflex is out of balance, think about this reflex area also covering jaw, teeth and throat - consider:

211

- Do they have any current pain in their mouth, jaw, throat or teeth?

- Are they prone to any conditions or infections in their mouth, jaw, throat or teeth?

- Do they hold tension in their jaw when they are stressed?

- Do they suffer with a dry mouth – perhaps when they are stressed?

- Are they aware if they grind their teeth at night?

Emotional prompts:

This is about what we take in and reject in communication terms.

- Are they speaking up and putting their view forward?

- Are they swallowing any situation because they believe they can't change it? Is there something they could do to change it?

- Are they able to express easily their core beliefs and ideas?

- Are they speaking their truths and values or someone else's?

The skin

Physical prompts:

- Do they have or have they ever had any skin problems?

- Do they have sensitive skin?

Emotional prompts:

This is all about integration of self to the outside world, which may or may not be difficult.

- Are issues getting under their skin?

- Are they irritated by something?

Index

213

215

Notes